Dr. Anne's

MAGIC-HAND Eating Plan

Also by Anne Seifert:

His, Mine and Ours: A guide to keeping marriage from ruining a perfectly good relationship, Macmillan Publishing Company, 1979. ISBN0026090309

The Intelligent Woman's Diet: The practical way to keep trim, relax, and stay well the rest of your life, Varnes Publishers, 1982. ISBN0943584019

All books can be ordered from the www.dranne.org website.

MAGIC-HAND® *Eating Plan*

Good Health, Happiness and Weight Control

***Anne Seifert**, M.P.H., Ph.D.*

Varnes ♑ Publishers
Seal Beach, California

Varnes Publishers
1562 Golden Rain Rd. 44G
Seal Beach, CA 90740-4938
varnes@adelphia.net

Library of Congress Control Number: 2004109772

Seifert, Anne.
MAGIC-HAND Eating Plan: good health, happiness and weight control

ISBN 0-943584-03-5

First Edition

Printed in the United States of America

MAGIC-HAND® Eating Plan

by Anne Seifert, M.P.H., Ph.D.

A nine point visual and mental training course

This book is divided into two sections: MANUAL and PRACTICE

Varnes Publishers ♑ Seal Beach, CA

Disclaimer--What this book will and will not do for you

This book is designed to provide information regarding healthy living and weight control. It is offered with the understanding that each person is different, and it is the responsibility of the individual to check first with a health professional if there is any concern that the advice included herein might not apply for a specific situation or medical condition.

Every effort has been made to make this a flexible and adaptable program since you can choose your own foods in each food group. You are urged to tailor this information to meet your individual needs.

The purpose of this book is to educate the reader about well-balanced nutrition and to provide a life long food-based portion-control program for weight loss and maintenance. Individual results may vary and there is no guarantee as to how much weight will be lost following this program. The course of instruction given will for most people improve their general nutrition, health, and foster gradual safe weight loss.

Simply stated, know your own body and use your common sense when changing lifestyle habits.

MAGIC-HAND®

Eating Plan

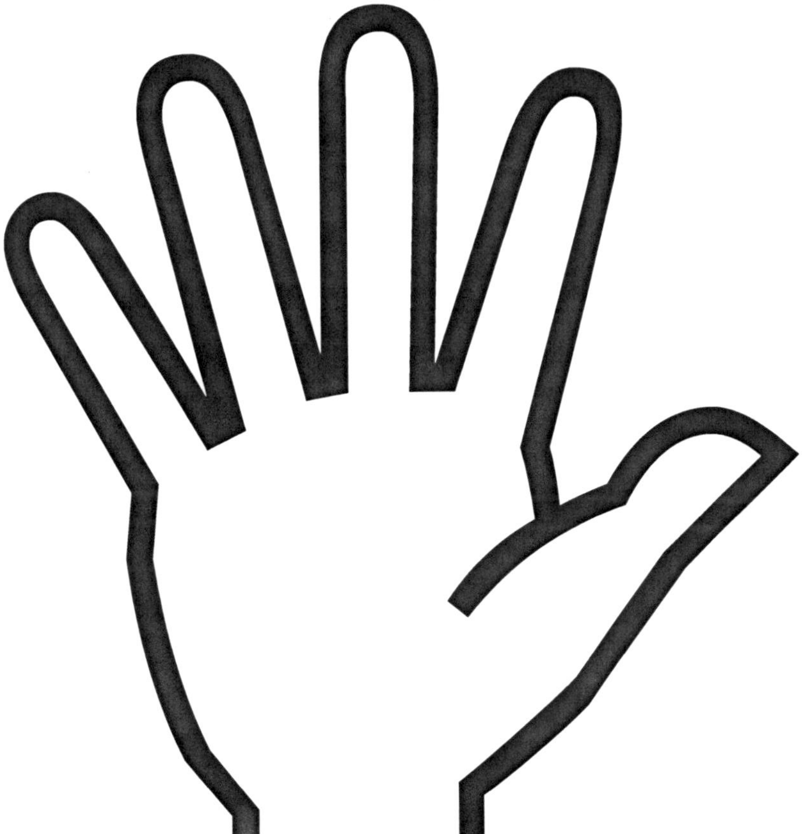

MANUAL

Introduction

Who couldn't use a "helping hand" when beginning major changes in lifestyle habits? It's even nice to have some support after you've achieved your goals, just to keep on track. We all have our good days and some bad days, but there's nothing like sharing our experiences as a way of helping ourselves and others along the way.

How to Use this Book

There are nine Points in this book and each Point has a chapter in the main MANUAL and a section with the same title in the PRACTICE. For example, Point 1 is called ***M***easure in the MANUAL and it relates to the section in the PRACTICE also called Point 1 ***M***easure. After you read a Point chapter in the MANUAL, if you'd like to do some self-exploration you can work on the corresponding PRACTICE Point.

While the MANUAL applies to everyone, the answers in the PRACTICE apply only to you.

If you want to get an overview of the program, then read the entire MANUAL first, and later answer the questions in the PRACTICE section.

Our goal is to promote healthy well-balanced eating for weight control and to make it easy and fun. In addition we want to encourage on-going support Circle Groups in every neighborhood. In these pages you will learn a way to keep your weight under control that is flexible and livable for a lifetime.

To the nines!

When I was a little girl I had an occasional bout of the hiccups. Once they started it seemed no matter what I did I couldn't get rid of them. My mother said, "Here, let me give you a little MAGIC". She filled a glass with water and told me to bend over and drink the water upside down. And guess what?

My hiccups disappeared.

*M*easure

● Point 1

Looking in the mirror glass

Anyone who is overweight and wants to lose weight knows the exquisite misery of facing the mirror and asking, "How did this happen to me?" Skirts and slacks are too tight. What you wore last summer to the beach doesn't look as good this year. The "camouflage" outfits travel forward from the back of the closet: loose blouses, big jackets, wrap-around skirts and the muu-muu dresses from years ago. You contemplate whether it's time to go on a diet. Your friends are losing weight right and left on liquid diets and two-week wonder wafers and you think that that's what to do. Just get the weight off. Then you can think about changing your lifestyle. Deep down inside though you know that the quick fixes are only temporary. (And your lifestyle probably won't change afterwards.) But, you know that if you want to keep your weight under control without going through sheer torture, the best and healthiest way to do it is by changing the way you eat, not for two weeks, but for every day of your life.

It may comfort you to know that you are not alone. Perhaps the reason we don't simply do what seems obvious and sensible--EAT LESS AND EXERCISE MORE-- is because it's just not as simple as it looks. Wearing a patch on your arm for 2 weeks to lose weight is easy. Foregoing the French fries is not. Skipping a meal is easier than counting calories. And what's wrong with finding another way out? Nothing, except that it's a temporary solution. You'll be gaining weight in a few months and tempted to buy more powdered drink mixes, more diet patches, more appetite suppressant candies and the like. On top of that, while you're gaining the weight back (because you didn't change your lifestyle), you won't feel good about yourself.

Getting your weight under control is a primary step towards good health and improved self-esteem. Cosmetic reasons are not the only reasons to lose weight. More important is the benefit to your health. Often it is only when you lose it that one realizes the importance of good health.

Almost all of us have had the experience of not being healthy and because of the way our minds work once we have recovered from our illness, we soon forget our misery. In the case of most chronic diseases we often feel just a little bit not well. It depends on the day or our mood. We just are not sick enough to do anything about it. It takes a major event to get our attention. When a severe episode of a life threatening illness strikes (like a heart attack) as we are carted into the Intensive Care Unit we resolve that from this day forward we will change our lifestyle habits, turn over a new leaf and live in a healthy way. After a close call we become thankful for every day and treasure what health remains.

Life threatening events and permanently disabling threats to our bodies have an "awakening" effect. You are never quite the same again and if fortunate, a lesson is learned, and you become a happier more thankful person who treasures what amounts to another chance. You become very motivated to change habits to preserve your health.

As an epidemiologist I learned that interventions can be implemented at very different levels often with the same result. For example, both the wearing of seat belts and driving at a reduced 55 miles per hour speed limit do save lives on the highway. The interventions are different, but each action works to reduce the highway death toll: one by reducing driver impact inside the car, and the other by reducing the number of automobile accidents in the first place.

From psychology I learned that emotional factors can override a person's own self-interest or other beneficial behavior. Self-sabotage and bad habits keep many of us from enjoying optimal health and happiness. And from nutrition I learned that there is much art to the science of eating. We are all specialized chemistry sets and what we eat sets the wheels in motion and keeps them going, but genetics play an important role as well. My experience in the health field has taught me that perhaps one of the most debilitating factors in the lives of most mobile "healthy" people is simply being overweight. In general it does not contribute to people's happiness and almost always it will accelerate any predisposing physical condition and make treatment for any physical problems more difficult. If there was one public health intervention I could recommend (especially for the United States) that would reduce premature death, physical ailments, surgery and its complications, and reduce the risk of most chronic diseases it would be for all people to eat properly, exercise moderately and keep their weight under control. If we could all do this, fewer hospitals would be built and our health costs would nose-dive. We would all be healthier people.

Most articles and books that are written by those trained in nutrition are based on sensible eating principles and focus on the ability of foods to meet nutritional (as opposed to weight loss) needs. However, when nutritionists do create reduced calorie diets for weight loss they become very complicated because there is tremendous focus on getting the right nutrients into the body. Therefore food tables are needed so that nutritionally similar foods can be grouped and interchanged with one another. The quantities must be limited and from a dietician's exacting point of view, they should be weighed or measured so that portions are comparable. Almost all well-balanced diets for weight loss include exchange tables, food groups, and measured quantities of food as caloric and/or nutritional equivalents. Sometimes these requirements are met in a liquid or powdered diet form, but even if they are nutritionally adequate they will probably fall short on roughage and other "non-essential" but desirable elements. The best diets use real foods that you can buy yourself in the supermarket.

Attempting to fill the gap are many commercial programs to help people lose and maintain their weight loss. I spoke with one graduate of such a program recently. She exclaimed how she lost 12 pounds on this nationally advertised program. I asked her if she now knew how to eat and she said, "Yes." What she learned was to eliminate almost all fat from her diet and to eat a diet containing very specific percentages of protein and carbohydrate. This program sold pre-packaged food which adhered to these stipulations. While she was in the program she simply ate the pre-packaged dinners. She did not die, but she was very hungry and her hair started to fall out. She was now on what she called "maintenance". She ate an orange and a banana for breakfast, a salad from a local salad bar for lunch with no butter or oil and for dinner she had a small portion of meat and a salad and a plain roll. Of course, she mentioned it was difficult for her to eat that way all the time, but she was trying. I told her she was on a "deprivation diet" and that it was quite understandable that she would be hungry. What she had learned from this program was to eliminate fat from her diet and to cut down on her portions. All very well and good, as long as she bought the pre-packaged meals. However, she still didn't know how to eat. And for maintaining weight loss on your own, you need to know how to eat. My prediction sadly is that she will eventually gain back all the weight that she lost. I am reminded of that proverb that basically states: If you give a man a fish he will again become hungry, but if you teach a man how to fish he need never be hungry again. In a sea of so many diet alternatives consumers are confused and want to believe that they will be successful with the doctor who prescribes pills and liposuction, the nutritionist who offers laborious recipes for reduced calorie menus and the packaged program "consultant" who advertises quick results and celebrity endorsements. All of these programs will work for a time. Unless you can maintain the weight loss on your own, however, you will continue to bounce from one weight loss scheme to another.

The least healthy way to lose weight is to fast, and then after that come the so-called "quick-fixes" like liquid diets and enforced starvation diets. The healthiest way to lose weight is through exercising and living a well-balanced eating lifestyle.

You will soon have the tool for staying healthy and staying slim. You are invited to learn a way of living and eating that can stay with you for all time through the pages of this book.

Finding the magic of a simple solution

The *MAGIC-HAND* Eating Plan began with my research to discover how healthy people stay healthy. It became clear to me after years of investigation that what we had always suspected was true: sensible eating, moderate exercise, eating breakfast, and sleeping 7 to 8 hours a night were associated with good health and well-being. If I could find a way to make nutritious well-balanced eating easy and exercise enjoyable, perhaps more people would do it.

I was able to distill the well-balanced, but often complicated diets recommended by nutritionists into one easy system-- the *MAGIC-HAND* Plan.

The principles that you will learn here work just like the magic that my mother used to help me get rid of my hiccups. What you will learn with some sleight of hand will enable you to stay slim for the rest of your life. That is a promise I can keep. What makes this system easy is that you do not need to count calories or weigh foods in order to eat nutritiously or to have a well-balanced diet.

This is a lifelong eating plan, a permanent way to keep the weight off. Once you learn the technique you will never be without your *MAGIC-HAND.*

From the start you will learn how to eat correctly and because it is a healthy diet, you just continue eating as instructed and include the foods you want. Its unique feature, and the basic tenet of the entire plan, is to use the hand to measure portion sizes. The hand becomes a visual estimator and measuring tool. This is what eliminates counting calories and using exchange tables. This is what separates the *MAGIC-HAND* Plan from all others making it a cinch to use. But, there's much more to it than that-- you can eat what you want, when you want, and what everyone else is eating. It's what's called natural magic. You eat the way a person eats who wants to stay slim without the feeling of being totally deprived. If you must, you could even eat French fries (although I'd hope for a better choice).

Weight loss is gradual and natural, averaging 1 to 2 pounds a week. You may lose more or less weight than that in a week depending on how overweight you are at the onset and on how grudgingly your body insists on holding on to fat. However, most people will reach their ideal weight within six months. If you only need to lose a few pounds it could happen in a month. Thereafter the weight loss is maintained forever by continuing to follow the *MAGIC-HAND* guidelines. It becomes a way of life for those who want to stay slim. And, like magic, the pounds vanish.

The *MAGIC-HAND* Eating Plan was developed to be easy, practical and so simple that anyone could follow its fun formula. At the same time it is a permissive diet, allowing you to still eat your favorite foods.

What you will learn is <u>how</u> to eat with a few simple hand tricks. The precise performance of these hand maneuvers will bring about the desired weight control outcome. And you will know what to eat. Each Point focuses on an aspect of weight control that will help you to maintain your ideal body weight. The eating plan itself is easy to follow and implement, but you will need to integrate exercise into your life as well. I believe that sharing with others helps to keep us motivated and suggest that after you read each chapter that you review and complete the exercises in the accompanying *MAGIC-HAND* Practice by yourself and/or in a Circle Group. Each Point in the PRACTICE is matched to the Point in the MANUAL. Use the PRACTICE to document your thoughts and record your insights. To get started (as you read the Point chapters ahead) write down everything you eat in the next three days-- that is, what you are really eating right now. Identify the food and quantity and time of day. Later we'll use that information to construct a new way of eating. Remember there are no right or wrong answers, so be honest. We will talk more about your style of eating later.

The *MAGIC-HAND* Plan will make those pounds disappear and, more importantly, will help you stay slim and healthy for the rest of your life.

Look terrific. Feel great. That's the result.

Tuning in to your numbers

To determine what is the best or ideal weight for yourself requires adequate self-knowledge. Very few people have <u>never</u> experienced the joy of being at a desirable weight. It <u>is</u> possible that you may have the so-called "fat gene" which means that you are more likely to accumulate fat than other people. It is well known that **where** fat accumulates on your body is an inherited characteristic. If you have a tendency to accumulate fat, like the alcoholic, you will need to subscribe to a life sentence of watchful eating to stay slim. (Take heart, you have company.)

Unless you were a chubby toddler, and an overweight youngster who never "outgrew" it, you can probably recall when you were really fit, and when you felt and looked good. If you cannot recall such a time, then I ask you to trust that it <u>is possible</u> for you to experience being slim and fit. By using your *MAGIC-HAND* you will reach the "ideal" weight for you-- you will have that experience. Natural weight loss that is gradual will bring you to the body weight that is your own best weight, and you will know this because it will be the body weight that you maintain as you continue to practice the *MAGIC-HAND*. You will be eating in the general range of about 1200-1500 calories a day which will initiate weight loss and then sustain the maintenance of your own unique ideal body weight!

For this reason there are two basic approaches one could take to determining ideal weight. It is important to know exactly what that number is because the scale can then validate your eating habits. You can either (1) determine an ideal target weight for yourself or, (2) not worry about a number-- let the *MAGIC-HAND* lead you to a final destination plateau weight. If you know what you want to weigh because that weight is when you looked and felt best, then claim that number as your ideal weight. Eventually-- whether you arrive at this number through the front door or back door-- you will have an ideal weight figure that you can maintain for the rest of your life. Whatever your weight is now, as you read this book, we will call your "starting weight". (Do you know how much you weigh?)

In addition you should establish an ideal dress size or pants size. You will also be maintaining the same size wardrobe for the rest of your life. Select a "target" outfit from your closet, one that you wish you could wear again and keep that dress or pair of slacks in mind as you lose weight. If you don't have an outfit in that size, buy one and keep it in your closet as an indicator, when worn, of your progress to date. You will see results month after month as the number on your scale declines and your target outfit gets roomier. Then one day you will be there, at your ideal weight. The scale will register the right number and the outfit you selected will fit. This signals the beginning of your lifelong commitment to the *MAGIC-HAND* Plan.

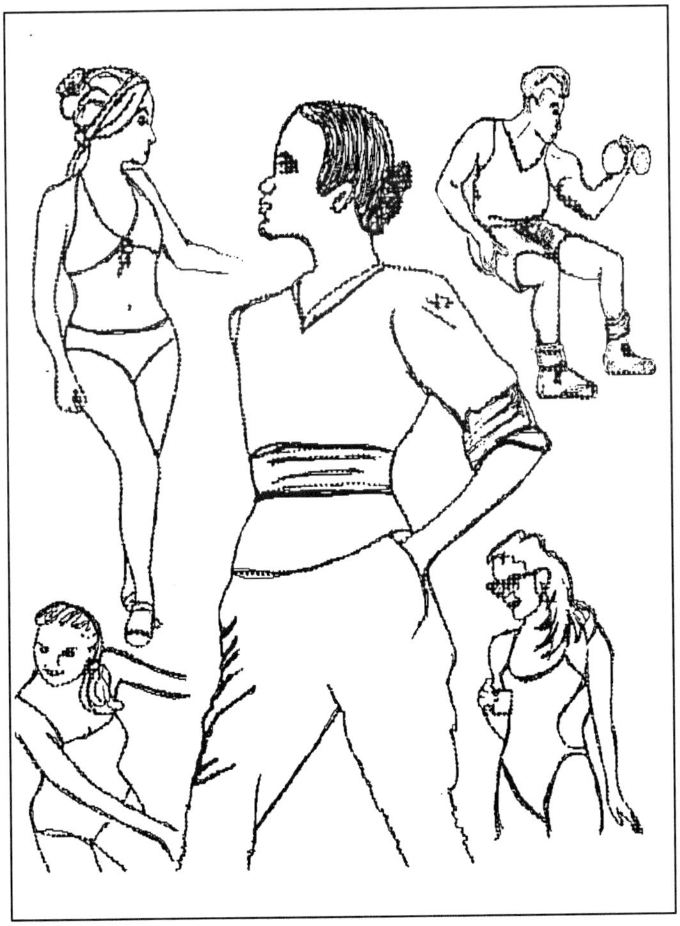

Finding the "right" body for me

Do you have a number in mind? What is your "ideal weight"? Think about it. When you have decided what that weight is, write the number down in the margin of this book. Then add two pounds to it, placing that number to the right of your ideal weight. Then subtract two pounds from your ideal weight and place that number to the left. So, for example, if your "ideal weight" is 128 pounds, you would have 126 on the left and 130 on the right. The range, 126-130 pounds, in this example, would be your "ideal weight range". You should strive to keep your weight within that range at all times. Few of us need to worry about going below our ideal weight. Because there are natural fluctuations in weight due to water intake and other factors, you need not worry as long as you stay within your ideal range. However, you'll want to stay as close to your exact target as possible. If you get to the top of your ideal weight range it is time to reevaluate your behavior. It's time to ask yourself: Have I strayed from the principles of the *MAGIC-HAND* eating? What happened? Did your *MAGIC-HAND* lose some control?

When you find the reason, correct yourself immediately. This is a warning signal that you MUST heed. By the same token any weight loss that brings you below your ideal weight range must be evaluated as well. It may signal some underlying physical condition requiring medical attention. You are to stay at your ideal healthy weight. If you fall two pounds below, be alerted and if you gain two pounds above, the warning bell should ring. You must be on constant guard and not take your previous weight loss for granted. After you become practiced in using your *MAGIC-HAND* you can become overly confident about your abilities. Because the eating plan is so comfortable and livable you may be deluded into thinking that you no longer need to count your portions. There's a temptation to start taking too many "liberties" with eating because you've been holding your ideal weight. Avoid the temptation to regress back to your old ways-- the lifestyle that helped you to gain the weight. You will discover just how much liberty you can take and it is for this reason that you are given the "warning signal" at a two-pound gain. Remember your ideal weight and your weight range and never allow yourself to get outside that range. This is the commitment you must make to yourself and it is lifelong if you want to enjoy optimal health and slim, trim results. Keep in mind that every body is different. You are the best judge of your desirable weight. (And if you are building muscle you could actually gain weight while your clothes get baggy.)

At the same time this is a very livable eating plan, so relax. You really will be able to make a lifelong commitment to it without tremendous suffering and deprivation.

Making a pact

To help you make this commitment I strongly urge that you implement the program just as I recommend. Besides determining your ideal weight and mentally visualizing yourself there, I want you to find a "buddy". This is someone who you can trust who will meet with you every month for a check-in. This person need not necessarily be using the *MAGIC-HAND* Eating Plan. You just need a reliable person who is willing to spend approximately one minute a month with you so that you can verbally tell him or her how much you weigh. This is very important. Your "buddy" is requested only to listen to your report and should not dole out advice or make any comments or suggestions or be critical in any way. This simple reporting requirement will keep you going and force you to be conscious of the fact that you are in control of your weight. Again, this requirement is lifelong. You never stop reporting once a month. Decide who would be a good person for you. Make it convenient for yourself and choose someone who is usually available either by phone or in person. (I "check-in" with my neighbor who I usually see anyway and who similarly gives me his report.) Select a person who is likely to be around for a while, so you do not need to keep replacing people.

Once you decide on the right person, contact your future "buddy", and ask if he or she would be willing to allow you to check-in with him once a month to report your weight (that's all). At first it will feel just a little uncomfortable to tell someone else what you really weigh. But, I cannot emphasize enough the importance of this little ritual. It will keep you on track. Just think of how proud you'll be when you can report your lower weight each month. And you can be even prouder reporting your weight month after month when it's within your ideal weight range.

Remember it is your weight that you report, not the number of pounds lost. The actual number that reads on your scale is what counts here. To that end, be sure that you have an accurate scale placed in a convenient spot perhaps in your bedroom or bath. Check the reading a few times to see if the type of flooring (carpet or linoleum) in your home affects the numbers. You want consistency and accuracy and if you can't get it with your present scale, please buy a new one. Be brave. Step on the scale and record what you get. This is an investment in your future, and you should view your scale as an item that will be with you for the long term. Get one that works. Because of slight variations in manufacture, it is best to always use the same scale when weighing-in each month. This should always be done on the same day of the month and early in the morning after urination. To repeat, your monthly weight reading should be done on the same scale, on the same day of the month, upon arising after you urinate, and without wearing clothes or shoes-- au natural.

Select a day or date of the month that will be easy for you to remember. Do not be concerned that there are unequal days in a month or that if you pick every second Sunday of the month as your weigh-in and report date, that the time intervals between recordings will be unequal. I guarantee that your weight loss will be unequal too and what matters is the trend. You should be gradually losing weight and leveling at your ideal weight. Since this date is a lifetime date, select a day that for whatever reason is easy for you to remember. On this date you will record your weight. It could be the seventeenth of every month or the first Sunday of every month. The only requirement is that it occurs every month and that it is easy for you to remember. You should then report the weight you recorded to your "buddy" as soon as possible.

Assuming that you have identified your ideal weight and calculated your ideal weight range, let's establish an easy record keeping system for each month. You will need a pen and a 3"X 5" lined index card.

On the first line of the card, left hand side, write your initials; on the right hand side put today's date. On the next line put your starting date (month, day, year) that will be your consistent time to weigh-in each month. Also write the day of the week on which that date falls. For example, your second line might read 03/06/YR (SA). Let’s say March 6th fell on a Saturday that year.) Each month you will record the date and day. After you write down the date, record your weight on that date. For example, 03/06 (SA): 143. This means that on your starting date, March 6th, a Saturday, you weighed 143 pounds. As you enter the data each month try to keep your entries in straight columns. That way, with a quick glance, you can see how you're doing. On the right side of the card on the same line as your starting weight, the second line, write your goal weight and range. For example, GOAL: 126-128-130. In this case your ideal weight is 128 pounds and your range, from low to high is 126 to 130 pounds. You can circle or underline your ideal weight so that it stands out. When you hit 130 pounds you will know that you are at the top of your ideal weight range. This index card procedure is illustrated in detail in the *MAGIC-HAND* Practice.

You might be wondering why you record your weight only at monthly intervals. While you are losing weight it may take a while for the scale to register the loss. If you weighed yourself every day you would see fluctuations up and down. You may weigh yourself as much as you wish if you can't stand the suspense, but only record your weight once a month on the card. The weight on the card is what counts. At times you may feel depressed and looking back at what you have accomplished is motivating and inspiring. It is also helpful to notice the times when you hit the top of your ideal weight range and then, to try to analyze what happened in your life at that time. After a while you will have a collection of index cards to document your weight loss and weight maintenance experience. Save them all. You may start to notice seasonal cycles and even times when you approach the bottom of your ideal range. It's not unusual for people sometimes to go below their ideal weight during the summer months (if they are increasing their exercise activity) and to hit the warning signal at the top after all the December holidays. These cards show your history of weight loss and gain patterns.

Well-balanced eating and natural weight-loss is our goal.

Your old actions bought you excess pounds and that's what needs to be changed. What we tend to forget is that people who have problems keeping their weight under control just cannot be given free rein in front of an "all you can eat" buffet. There are people who can eat without overeating. They are slim. They are often aware of when they are hungry and when they are not. Somehow they know when to stop. If we were like these slim people, we would not have this problem! But, we're not, and it is necessary to recognize that fact.

Accept the truth about yourself. You have suffered from an inability to eat in a way that will allow you to maintain your ideal weight. It is unlikely that you will ever be able to eat without being conscious of your intake because your bodily mechanisms, either physiological or psychological or both, are not functioning towards keeping your ideal body weight. They are out of kilter. And if you continue to abuse yourself with starvation type diets, your condition will worsen. It is time to take healthy action, to correct your eating behavior and to commit for a lifetime. I wish I could tell you that there was an instant reversal, but there is not. This book will bring results, but only if you follow the principles of the *MAGIC-HAND*. You have the condition of being overweight. It is not a national disaster. You have a lot of company in the same boat. You can be thankful that the situation is indeed correctable.

The pill that is so difficult to swallow is that the permanent correction requires commitment for a lifetime because you don't know, never learned and were not brought up to eat correctly. New habits must replace the old. This will be the learning of a new act for you.

At the next Point you will learn how to eat for the rest of your life. So, let's get on with the show!

You're on your way!

Go to PRACTICE M1 now.

*A*pportion

● Point 2

Dealing the *MAGIC-HAND*

Instead of one magic potion, you have the opportunity now to learn a set of principles comprised of healthy eating basics to achieve weight loss. What you will learn in this chapter is actually a re-learning of what you probably already "know" and suspect is true: that eating regular balanced meals throughout your life is healthy, and the tried and true way to permanent weight loss.

Nevertheless I can understand the desire to want to believe in fairy tales and quick solutions. I'll never forget the woman who came running over to me at one of my first *MAGIC-HAND* seminars. She was so excited and enthused about this new diet and asked, "Tell me, where is the spot that I press on my hand to lose weight?" She was educated, intelligent and "knew" better, but still wanted to dream that maybe this would be an instant solution; maybe this would be a trick that would work. Maybe this time she could just press the magic spot on her hand and lose ten pounds. Don't we all wish? It is difficult to face the pain and reality that being overweight means that at some point we just ate too much. Truly it is not the end of the world and wonderfully it is correctable through healthy balanced eating.

You must simply decide whether you want to engage in a yo-yo struggle of weight loss and weight gain, **OR** whether you want to invest in modifying your lifestyle by altering your eating habits. Both scenarios apply for a lifetime. In the first solution your normal eating is a weight-gain diet and it is corrected by a usually severe and restrictive diet or fasting episode. The cycle repeats itself. In the second solution your normal eating is corrected in order to maintain the desired weight. The cycle is broken. The correction requires re-education. Your choice. In this book you will get the special knowledge you need to break that lifetime yo-yo cycle. Be assured that this *MAGIC-HAND* has been tested and that it is easy to follow and to live with for the rest of your life. Others have done it and you can too. Assuming you have decided that healthy weight loss is preferable to any other alternative, you have made the right choice. How do we start? We start by recalling an earlier time when we were in grammar school and our teacher told us about proper eating and good nutritional habits. To gain back this fundamental knowledge that we may have lost over the years, a review of the basic nutritional concepts underpinning a well-balanced diet is required reading. In the pages ahead you will relearn what may seem quite elementary, but it is also important because it provides the foundation for balanced meal planning.

Your first homework assignment

Select three consecutive days of your life (if you can remember the previous three days' meals, that's fine), and write down everything you eat, and the time of day. If you are involved in some physical exercise also include the activity and time of day. Be honest, after all this record is for your eyes only. This nutritional diary will establish your baseline and identify some of the foods you like to eat on a regular basis. As you learn the *MAGIC-HAND* it will have more meaning to you and you will be better able to judge how to reconstruct your present way of eating. You will need three separate sheets of lined paper for Day 1, Day 2 and Day 3 (or use the form below).

For 3 days, please write down: the *Time, Food Item, and Quantity.*

Day 1	Day 2	Day 3
Breakfast	**Breakfast**	**Breakfast**
Lunch	**Lunch**	**Lunch**
Dinner	**Dinner**	**Dinner**
Snacks:	**Snacks:**	**Snacks:**
Total Calories=	Total Calories=	Total Calories=

(activity)	*(activity)*	*(activity)*

ACTIVITIES? What did you do to "burn up" calories each day and how long did you do it?

If you can find the calories on the package of the food item you consumed, or you have an approximate idea or access to a calorie book, add the number of calories for each day.

Basic training begins

Do you remember the charts our teachers would display showing us the Basic Food Groups? As youngsters we were taught that in order to balance a diet, foods from these various food groups had to be included in our daily meals. But as adults many of us have forgotten the basics: in order to balance a diet, to make it nutritionally sound, we must eat from a variety of food groups. If a diet does not include foods from these various groups on a daily basis it is probably unbalanced, and that means unhealthy!

Any diet proposing that you eat as much as you want of only one food to the exclusion of all others is inherently dangerous. You may lose weight initially on a poor diet because psychologically you can only eat so many bananas or pineapples in one day. Eventually, however, your body "hungers" for what it needs and it is not unusual for people to gain all their weight back plus some after a deficient diet because now the body has experienced nutrient deprivation and reacts by "storing" energy to increase survival odds. Wouldn't you do the same thing? If suddenly you no longer had all of the items you needed, you would make sure to buy twice as much the next time. Many Americans are on chronic deprivation diets while their bodies are busy storing or adding fat. This doesn't make sense. The deprivation is nutritional but the body's compensation is caloric. The body reasons that if it eats enough food--whatever is available--it is more likely to find the missing nutrients. This may be a good strategy in the jungle. Translating to modern times this means that people who are on extremely low-calorie diets (less than 1,000 calories a day) are simply not meeting their needs for important nutrients and because of this severe deprivation they will later stock up with calories. I guarantee that if you eat well-balanced meals, not only will you look and feel better and lose weight, but you will be astonished by how much you can eat. Your body will not be signaling physiological nutritional hunger. If you experience hunger it is more likely to be of the psychological variety common in binge eaters (to be addressed later).

The habits we have formed as adults have contributed to whatever shape we now find ourselves. If you want to break the cycle of degenerative bad health and weight gain, then you must be willing to change your habits. On this plan you will quickly learn what food groups you tend to favor at the expense or exclusion of others.

There are six *MAGIC-HAND* Food Groups: (1) Milk & Dairy, (2) Fruits, (3) Carbohydrates, (4) Protein, (5) Oils & Fats, and (6) Vegetables. In order to use this plan you must know what foods fall into the various food groups. Most people know, for example, that an apple is a fruit--but how do you know if kidney beans are a carbohydrate or a protein? Sometimes a food can actually belong in more than one group. The kidney bean for example is considered an excellent source of protein (especially for vegetarians) and could substitute for meat or fish. It is also a complex carbohydrate, and could be used in meal planning as a substitute for bread, cereal or pasta.

If you already know what foods belong in these groups you can skip this section. Here is a brief review of our SIX FOOD GROUPS:

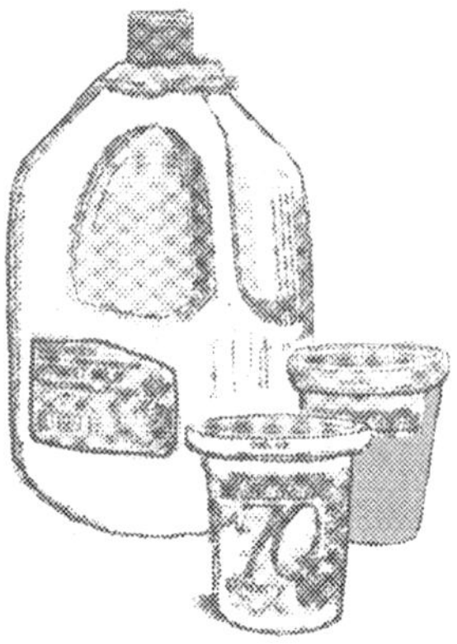

(1) MILK & DAIRY

Milk is generally considered an almost perfect food because it supplies protein for tissue building, calcium for bone growth, and riboflavin for the metabolism of amino acids. The Milk Food Group's main nutrient contribution is calcium, protein and riboflavin. Dairy products most people are familiar with are buttermilk, yogurt, cheese, and yes, ice cream! Look for the low-fat cheese and milk products. Women should perhaps be more conscious of their need to include milk in the diet to insure an adequate intake of calcium for the prevention of osteoporosis. It is a false saving if you are worried about calories and skip milk. In the portion sizes we recommend you will not gain weight and for women, especially over 40, calcium reserves are important in order to curtail bone loss. While milk is considered by some to be an almost "perfect" food, it does not supply adequate amounts of Vitamin C. And that is why we need:

(2) FRUIT

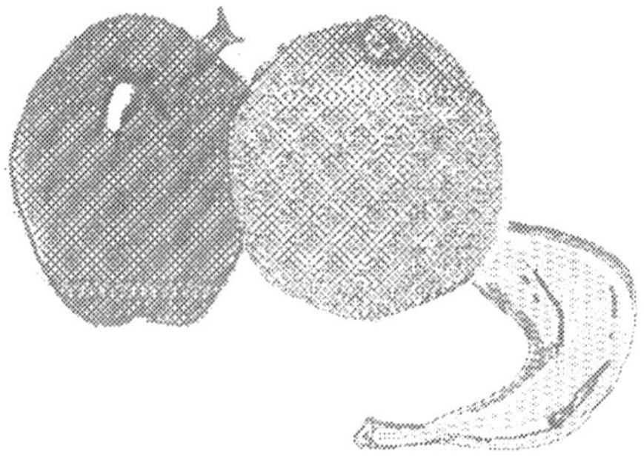

Vitamin C is the only vitamin not stored in our bodies, so it must be constantly replenished. Fruits also are wonderful for supplying roughage and keeping our sweet tooth in check.
In fact this may be why we humans have a sweet tooth--so that we would eat fruit! Unfortunately many of us got carried away with sweets, and have been paying the price ever since. So, even though many nutritionists lump the vegetable and fruit food group together because they both are good sources of vitamin C, in the *MAGIC-HAND* Eating Plan fruits and vegetables are separated because fruits are quite different calorically from vegetables. With the *MAGIC-HAND* you can get your sweet fix from an apple, or an orange, or a peach or some strawberries.

The next three food groups are labeled as Carbohydrate, Protein and Oil. Almost all foods contain some of each of these nutrients. Foods relatively high or considered a good quality source of that component are classified in that food group.

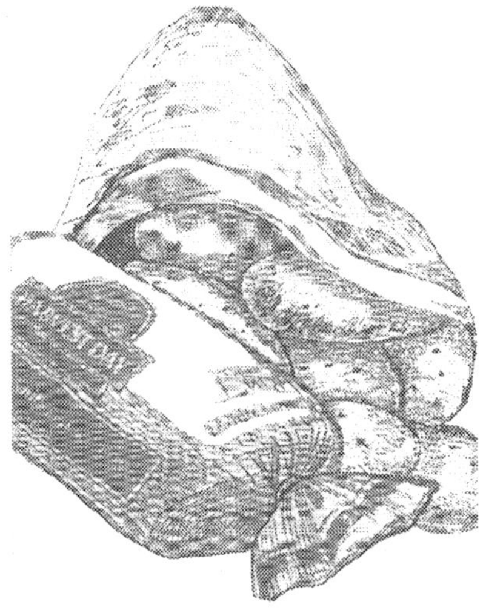

(3) CARBOHYDRATE

This food group refers to the starchy carbohydrates including grains, breads and cereal products as well as rice and pasta. Besides supplying "quick energy", additional riboflavin, niacin and iron are gained from these foods. Of course, the more natural the product and the less refined, the more likely the food is to contain other trace vitamins and minerals as well. And the less refined the food, the more roughage also. We recommend complex carbohydrates for weight reduction over foods containing simple sugars. Potatoes and corn are also included in this category (rather than in vegetables) because of their high (complex) carbohydrate content. These complex carbohydrates when combined with legumes also supply quality protein.

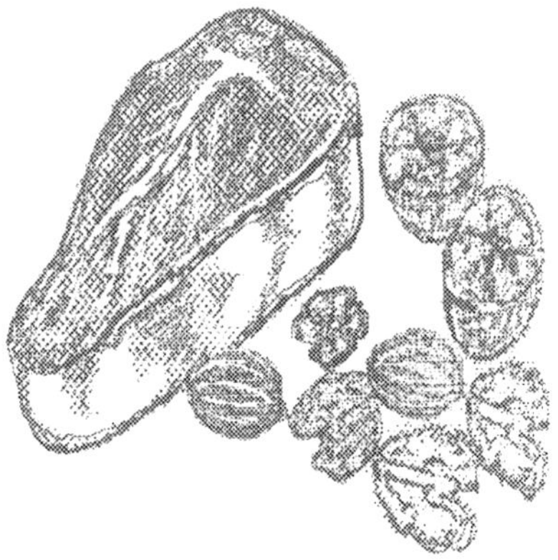

(4) PROTEIN

When most people think of protein they think of meat, and many nutritionists feel that the "best" proteins are animal proteins because their essential amino acid composition is closest to that of human protein. (It is also true that animal proteins generally contain more fat than vegetable proteins so there is a trade-off.) However, to utilize animal protein fully, plant protein is also necessary. Vegetarians can adequately meet their protein requirements by food combining but still they may have difficulty supplying enough Vitamin B-12, which is in short supply in the vegetable world. For the B-complex vitamins the best sources are beef, pork, lamb, fish and poultry. Good quality protein is also found in eggs, nuts, lentils, dry beans, peas and legumes. We need protein for muscle and tissue building and repair.

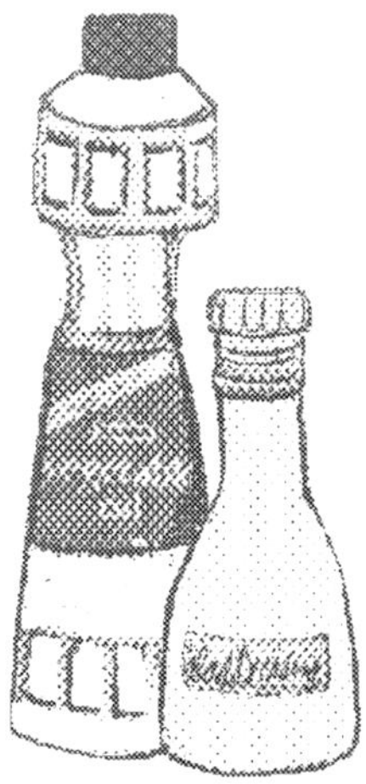

(5) OILS AND FATS

You may be wondering why I have added oils and fats as a food group. Clearly they are non-essential, and it is possible (but not advisable) to totally eliminate them from your daily menu. There is one important reason for their inclusion. Here experience has been my teacher. While you are losing weight there are two psychological saboteurs that can really get you down. One is the feeling of deprivation ("I can't have") and the other is the feeling of being hungry ("I want to eat all the time"). Oils and fats are included because usually people used to eating butter will feel deprived without a pat of butter on their toast, but more importantly fats are the last food to be digested in the stomach, so the feeling of being satisfied with your meal, with not being hungry, lasts longer when you include some fat at each meal. How much fat you should include will be discussed soon.

(6) VEGETABLES

On a plan to lose weight, vegetables are your best friends. They do so much and for so little. Not only do they provide vitamins and minerals and roughage, but they are filling, satisfying, tasty and contain hardly any calories! The Vegetable food group includes green ones like broccoli, spinach, and lettuce, and the so-called yellow ones like carrots and winter squash, rich in vitamin A.

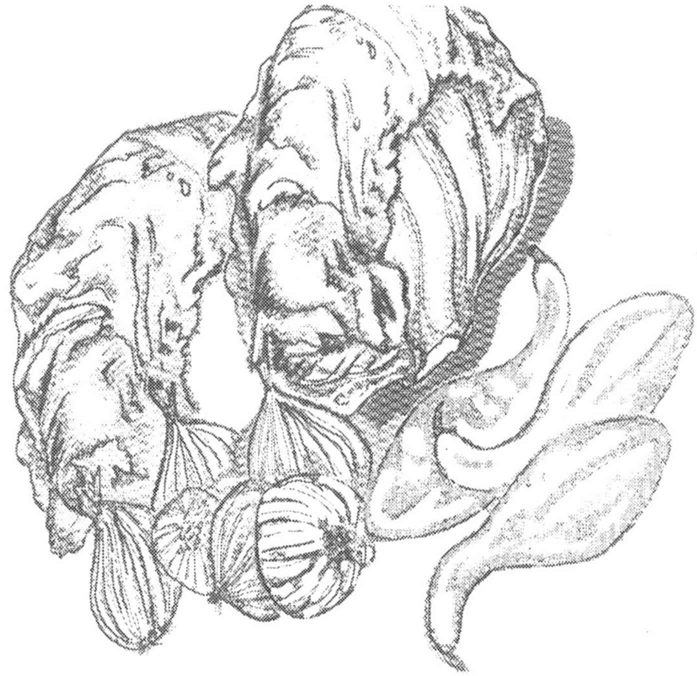

You will recognize that all well-balanced diets are basically the same. That's because they **are** including all the food groups. To summarize, the food groups to be included in your daily eating are:

* Milk and dairy products
* Fruits
* Carbohydrates
* Proteins
* Oils
* Vegetables

It sounds like a lot of food, but just to meet your body's basic nutritional requirements about 1200 calories (of the "right" foods) would be minimal. Fewer calories than that could actually stress your body and contribute to nutritional deficiency. If you want to lose weight, changing the quality of your diet will help, but it is not enough. Portion size must be limited, and exercise increased. Of these six food groups, only one food group needs no restriction. Can you guess which one? Vegetables are so low in calories and so filling that you can eat as many as you'd like and still not gain weight. So, there are five food groups requiring portion-size restriction and these are called the FIVE FINGER FOOD GROUPS. And you thought the finger-palm trick was used only by magicians! Well, it's for dieters too--on the *MAGIC-HAND* Eating Plan.

Now you need to know, "How much?" What follows is **some** magic--some sleight of hand!

Your hand is the tool

In order to make following a healthy well-balanced diet practical and easy we need to establish a standard serving size that would work across all food groups. This would eliminate the use of scales for weighing foods and reference tables. The tool that I discovered that is so practical and (literally) so handy to use is the "natural" server of man— the tool we used before we invented the knife and fork. It is nature's most natural measure. Our early forebears ate unprocessed nuts, fruits and seeds from the palms of their hands.

The measurer is your own hand! But don't envision yourself dipping your hand into cooked foods. Your hand does not replace a knife and fork. All you really need in order to follow this diet is various parts of your hand to **gauge portions**. You will learn to **visualize** the correct portion-size. This requires **your** judgment. Food is handled only when it is natural to do so. (For example, holding an apple.) Your hand can also be placed over the food. (For example, in gauging the size of a steak.) And you will keep track of your food groups by using your fingers to count the FIVE FINGER-PALM FOODS. Of course what's in your mind--the desire, motivation, and discipline to create the body you the want--is essential.

Using your own body part as a measurer has historical significance. The "hand" is a unit of length originally defined as the width of a man's hand from the little finger to the thumb. Units of various lengths known as hand or palm where used by the ancient Egyptians, Hebrews, Greeks, Romans and others. Because there was no better way, people used parts of their bodies to measure things. The "palm" was the width of four fingers and a "yard" was the length from the end of your nose to the end of your hand. These measures were always available and easy to use. The inch was the length of a man's thumb. As the Romans marched all over Europe they left behind common units of length. With the ability to measure precisely, the hand became standardized at 4 inches (10.16 centimeters) from a statute decreed by Henry VIII of England. In the recipe for his Crepes Suzettes, Henri Charpentier, the cook for Albert, the Prince of Wales, describes placing the amount of butter in a skillet as one joint of your thumb.

Moreover, the hand's breadth is a measure still used today to measure the height of horses from the ground to the withers. In linear measure the "hand" is four inches. And your own hand is the tool we will use on the *MAGIC-HAND* Plan. (But you will not be eating like a horse!)

The hand is used as the measurer for portion or serving size. You literally have a helping hand. We can envision what would fit into our cupped hand or what would fit under the outline of the palm of our hand. Rather than to rely on a technical instrument to give us a reading we can use one of our senses--sight. We can look at a portion size and determine if it is the same size as a specific part of our hand. The advantage to this measuring tool over all others is that you always have it with you (convenience) and the size of your hand is naturally proportioned to your body and bone structure. Everyone has a different size hand and it is the right size for him or her! As you might expect, the smaller the person, the smaller the hand. The size of your hand also, in almost all cases, follows very closely to the portion sizes recommended on those voluminous lists of exchange tables. We will also use the hand as a measurer and as a reminder of what foods to include at each meal. It governs only the FIVE FINGER FOODS that need to be controlled in order to achieve successful weight loss and management: Milk, Fruit, Carbohydrate, Protein, and Oil.

So let's take a look at your hand. Focus on your palm and imagine that in the palm you could fit an apple, or a small roll or a hamburger patty. For example, my palm measures about 3" X 4" and when cupped would hold about a quarter to a half-cup of something. These palm-portion helpings are correct amounts to eat for losing weight and coincidentally in most cases are very close to the serving amount recommended on the "official" food group exchange tables. No calculating, no weighing foods: you can gauge portion-size by just imagining what would fit in your own palm! Could it be any easier to correctly size a portion? The size of your own hand is very concrete, very exact, and not really subject to interpretation. Something either fits in your palm or it does not. (Loose interpretations are tantamount to cheating or taking extra amounts on this diet.)

Seeing Fingers

Let's look at your hand again. We'll study the fingers this time. O.K., five on each hand. And five food groups that need monitoring. Again, they are: Milk & Dairy, Fruit, Carbohydrate, Protein and Oil & Fats. So now you know that for cheese, fruit, cereals, breads and other baked goods, and meat, poultry and fish, and butter, fats and oils that it is the size of your own hand--palm and fingers--that governs the portion size.

If you can, please follow these instructions with me and actually do what I say. Remember you will be visualizing the foods that you eat in relationship to your hand size. When practical you can actually place the food in your hand.

Turn your palm-up making a Hi-Five with the fingers of your right hand facing towards you. Starting with your pinky assign a word to each finger. Your pinky is "My", the next finger is "Fingers", the middle finger is "Count", the index finger is "Portions" and the thumb is "Offering". Looking at each individual digit of your hand, from pinky to thumb, assign one word to each and say aloud, "My Fingers Count Portions Offering". This phrase will help you to remember the food groups and the fact that their portion size is governed by your hand: Milk, Fruit, Carbohydrate, Protein, and Oil.

By now you may have noticed that the first letter of each word in the phrase "**M**y **F**ingers **C**ount **P**ortions **O**ffering " corresponds to the first letters of the FIVE FINGER FOODS. To finish the sentence add **V**ariety (to include Vegetables). Say this chant aloud to remember the food groups:

"**M**y	**F**ingers	**C**ount	**P**ortions	**O**ffering	**V**ariety"
Milk	**F**ruit	**C**arbohydrate	**P**rotein	**O**ils	**V**egetables

While you hold this book in your left hand keep looking at your right hand, palm facing you. As you can see there are four fingers directly above your palm. These four fingers represent the four food groups--Milk, Fruit, Carbohydrate and Protein--and serving sizes for these are measured using the palm of your hand. The food should fit within the parameters of your palm and you can either hold the food in your hand or visually match your palm to the food portion. The helpings are called palm-portions.

The only finger we haven't discussed is your thumb representing the Oil food group. Look again at your hand. The serving size for Oils and Fats is governed by your thumb size. You "only" get a very small portion.

You may notice we did not include Vegetables as a food group monitored by the hand. And that is because you can eat as many vegetables as you please on the *MAGIC-HAND* Plan. Portions are not controlled. But to remind yourself, look at your hand again and see that between the index finger and the thumb is an open "V", and that is for Vegetables! Memorize this chant while studying your hand for the next three minutes. "My Fingers Count Portions Offering Variety." Look at your fingers and that open "V". Say "My Fingers Count Portions Offering Variety" as you go from pinky to thumb. Look at the fingers above the palm governing Milk, Fruit, Carbohydrate and Protein and visualize a food item from each food group fitting into your palm. (In Appendix C you will find a list of foods that fall under each Finger-Palm category.) Go to your refrigerator and look for foods you could actually pick up and hold in the palm of your hand. Notice how one egg seems to fit perfectly in the palm of your hand. (That would be 1 Protein.) Then look at your thumb and visualize an Oil or for example, a pat of butter the size of the first joint of your thumb! When you can clearly visualize these portions then you will know the serving size of foods from the HI-FIVE food groups. You will never be in doubt as to how much food to put on your plate. Look at your palm, visualize the portion, and serve yourself. However, there are a few refinements you should know about. In actual practice questions arise, "How thick should the portion be?" The portion should be no thicker than your thumb held sideways with the nail facing you. (My thumb held sideways measures 3/4 in.)

And some foods are better suited to sizing and visualization in a cupped palm. For example, a small tangerine would fit nicely in your cupped palm. But, "How do I measure a liquid?" If you could hold a liquid in your cupped palm, about how much would it hold? Depending on your palm size it would be between 1/4 to 1/2 a cup of liquid. That's the basic idea. Use your palm as a measurer for the four food groups represented by the fingers above the palm and, depending on the food, either cup the palm or use the hand's breadth and thumb thickness as a measure. Either hold the food in your hand or visually estimate the fit.

The Oils food group includes butter, margarine, mayonnaise and cooking and salad oils. When oils and fats are liquid use the whole thumb (about 1 Tablespoon) as a portion size. When the oil or fat is solid, measure to the first thumb joint. (See Appendix A for specific amounts.) Because these foods are very high in calories the portion-size is very small, no larger than your thumb to the knuckle joint or the whole thumb. That means that on your palm-size slice of bread (no thicker than your thumb) you could have a thumb knuckle's worth of butter!

The FIVE FINGER FOOD helpings are controlled by the size of the palm and thumb of your own hand. You need never leave home without it! And once you actually practice this system it will be difficult to look at food servings any other way.

Creating your MAGIC-HAND

Did you notice the drawing of the hand on the cover of this book? It is now time for you to create your own *MAGIC-HAND.* This will be your own personalized hand that will have the power to govern your actions so that you eat correct portions from all the FINGER FOOD GROUPS.

<u>Apparatus:</u>

You will need some materials: Get an 8 1/2" X 11" thick sheet of paper, a good drawing pencil or pen and five approximately penny-sized round magnets (available sometimes at hardware or craft stores). Or use the sample page in PRACTICE Appendix D. You can make your own magnets simply by cutting out equal-size sections from any flat-type business or promotional card magnet.

<u>Procedure:</u>

Place the sheet of paper on a flat table surface and put your left hand, palm down on the sheet of paper. Place your hand so that there is enough room between the fingers to draw around them. Then take your pen and trace your left hand palm down. (Your pinky should be on the left and thumb on the right.) Above each finger write the name of the food group that belongs there. (Use the book cover as a model.) Darken the "V" area between your index finger and thumb so that you will remember that this open area means unlimited vegetables. Now draw a broken circle in the palm of your hand so that you will remember to use the palm-size. Divide each finger into three joints, and number each finger including the thumb starting at the top, 1, 2, and 3. This sheet should be attached to a metal surface (refrigerator, file cabinet-whatever) and the magnets placed inside the circle. Read on and you will see how to use your *MAGIC-HAND* to control your eating.

Now you know how many food groups you should include in your daily menu and how to control portion size. But, is that all the food you get? One portion of each of the FIVE FINGER FOODS? Fortunately for those of us who like to eat, the answer is "No". You get three hand or palm-portions from each of the FIVE food groups <u>every day</u>: 3 Milks, 3 Fruits, 3 Carbohydrates, 3 Proteins, and 3 Oils. Looking at it another way your daily menu consists of 15 *MAGIC-HAND* FINGER-PALM portions. (Vegetables are unlimited.)

Every time you eat, you must move the magnet on the corresponding finger food group. And, every portion is sized by your palm and/or thumb.

See Appendix D at the end of the PRACTICE section for a summary of the above instructions and a template for your drawing.

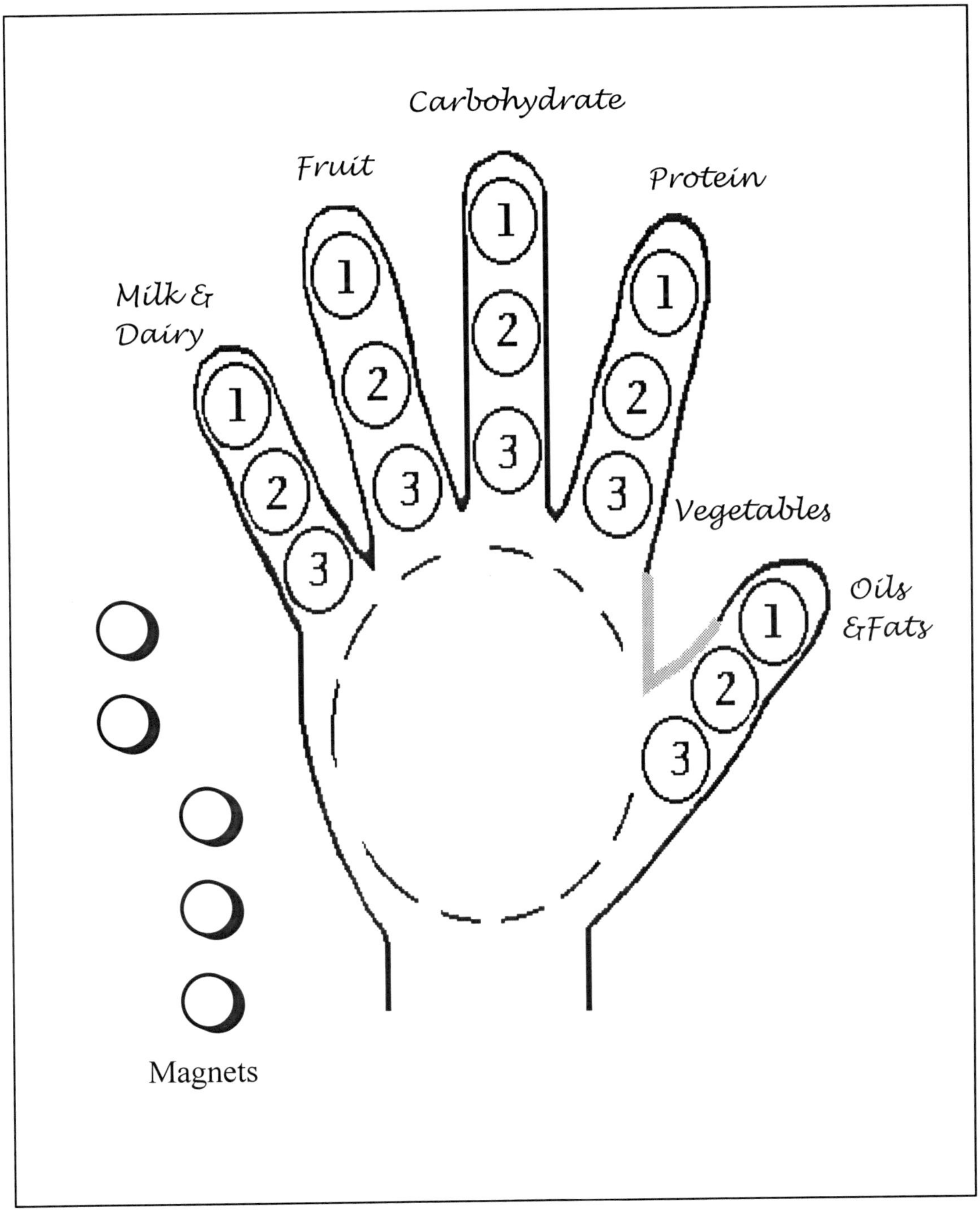

Your MAGIC-HAND!

How you want to distribute these servings over the day is your choice. In this way you could arrange to have a mid-morning and mid-afternoon snack. Here is a <u>*sample menu*</u> of what one day on the *MAGIC-HAND* Eating Plan could include:

Meal	***Quantity***	***Food Group***
Breakfast		
	cupped-palm grapefruit	1 Fruit
	palm-size bread slice	1 Carbohydrate
	1 egg	1 Protein
	1 thumb-joint butter /marg.	1 Oil
Snack:	1/4 cup yogurt /cupped-palm	1 Milk
Lunch		
	2 T. tuna fish /cupped-palm	1 Protein
	1 plate salad greens	1 Vegetable
	1 thumb dressing	1 Oil
	palm-size bread	1 Carbohydrate
Snacks:	1 cupped-palm size apple	1 Fruit
	1 palm-size slice cheese	1 Milk
	Carrot sticks	1 Vegetable
Dinner		
	palm-size chicken breast	1 Protein
	steamed broccoli	1 Vegetable
	1/2 cup (cupped-palm) of cream soup	1 Milk
	cupped-palm brown rice	1 Carbohydrate
	1 thumb-joint butter	1 Oil
	sliced palm-size peach	1 Fruit

TOTAL: 3 Milks, 3 Fruits, 3 Carbohydrates, 3 Proteins, 3 Oils

15 MAGIC-HAND servings: 3 servings from each Finger Food Group.

plus unlimited Vegetables

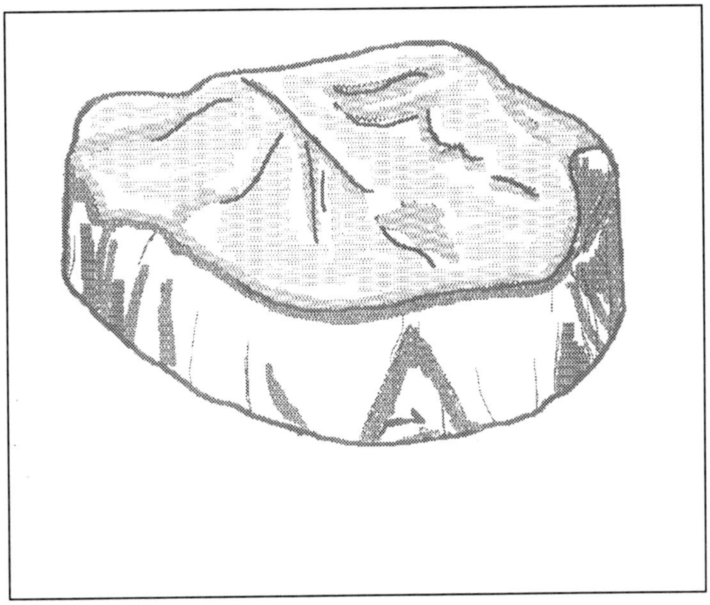

A portion that would fit in the palm of your hand!

Review the portions on the previous sample menu and imagine these quantities fitting into your hand. Some you could actually hold in your hand and others would be gauged by holding your hand near the food. As you review the sample menu, move the magnets on your personal *MAGIC-HAND* sheet to correspond to the foods that are eaten for breakfast, lunch and dinner. You will have one magnet for each finger or each food group. Start with breakfast placing a magnet on the number 1 for the correct food group finger and go through the meals, moving each magnet until all five magnets reach the number 3. This means you are through with the day's allotment of food. The next day you start all over again with all the magnets in the circle of the palm of the hand.

This is the technique you will use with your personalized *MAGIC-HAND* to give you the power to lose weight and keep it off. Think of it this way: you have a total of 15 chits a day- 12 palm-portions and 3 thumb-portions. The palm-portions can be flat and no thicker than your thumb or rounded and visually fit in the palm of your hand. The thumb-portions can be solid or liquid oils and visually sized by your thumb. Milk, Fruit, Carbohydrate and Protein Food Groups are always in palm-portions. Oils and fats are always in thumb-portions. Vegetables are always as much as you want. Got it? Imagine that you are "grounded", locked in your room, or that you are confined to a sailboat with limited supplies, and that you are given only 15 chits a day for your meals. How will you spend them?

Now make your own menu including the foods from each food group that you like to eat. In the corresponding Practice section you can create your own menus and list the foods you like under each Food Group heading. Remember there is no portion limitation for the Vegetable Food Group. On this *MAGIC-HAND* Eating Plan you will lose weight, preferably at a rate of 1 to 2 pounds a week, but if you are more than ten pounds overweight you can expect to lose even more every week. Once you have reached your ideal weight, then you can maintain that weight forever on a maintenance schedule.

The Golden Mean

In nature rainfall occurs at uneven intervals. One month's rainfall may be quite different from the next month's. Yet, on average, regions of the country are able to establish a general rainfall pattern for the year. Mother Nature tends to supply what is needed but She does so without concern for equally spaced or parceled rainfall. Mother Nature relies on the law of averages to keep this planet going. So, even if in one year the rainfall is below average, the next year might bring floods. In much the same way, the animal kingdom also survives. Sometimes it is feast and sometimes it is famine, but, on average, there is enough food to at least mature and produce a next generation. Fortunately for us, we humans have greater control over our environment and do not need to suffer extremes. Nevertheless to meet our bodies' nutritional requirements we do rely on the law of averages. We store many of the nutrients we need for healthy functioning in our cells, in our blood, and in our organs. Foods supply what we need, but not consistently, and depending on what stresses we encounter not always in the correct amount. However, on average, we are getting what we need from our foods to keep ready reserves and function well on a daily basis.

The *MAGIC-HAND* Eating Plan was designed allowing free-choice of foods in all food groups. Certainly the foods in each food group are not exactly the same, not nutritionally or calorically. However, most of the foods in a food group do supply common nutrients. Where these foods can differ more significantly is in caloric content. The emphasis here is on portion control and not calorie counting. As in nature the law of averages becomes operative. If you use palm-portions and vary your diet you will be eating different foods, some with more calories than others. Not all fruits, for example, are equal in calories even though they would fit in the palm of your hand. For example, a palm full of strawberries would have fewer calories than a palm full of grapes. The rule to be followed (if you are calorie-conscious) is that each palm-portion should be approximately 100 calories or less. Usually this upper limit is automatically controlled by the palm-portion size or will eventually average to 100 calories or less, so there is no reason to count calories. Just for your information, in the example I gave of strawberries and grapes, a half-cup of strawberries would be 29 calories and a half-cup of grapes would be 51 calories--both well under 100 calories. Most people could hold this amount of these fruits in their cupped palm. The important tenet to remember is not how many calories you are eating, but whether the portion fits in the palm of your hand. This is the only rule you need to follow. Do not worry about the calories!

Most refined foods are very calorie dense (with low nutrient density). For losing weight quickly we recommend that you avoid the "calorie dense" foods, even if they fit in the palm of your hand. But when you have reached your goal weight then you can begin to include more "calorie dense" foods if you wish, still fitting in the palm of your hand, without going off the Plan. Nutrient dense foods, however, are much preferred and healthier. In general if you avoid the foods that contain high concentrations of any refined sugars you will be eating less calorie dense, more natural foods. For very fast weight loss stay strictly with nutrient dense foods. However, if the situation arises where this is unavoidable or you simply "must" have some very calorie dense food, rather than to feel deprived, I recommend that you have a palm-portion to satisfy your craving or psychological hunger. You will still lose weight because you are on the *MAGIC-HAND* Plan and the law of averages will eventually work. If sometimes you eat foods that are calorie dense and at other times you eat foods that are less dense, eventually the lower calorie foods will compensate for the higher calorie foods, and on average, you will be holding a steady weight-loss course. However, if you want to lose weight quickly, do not take too many detours!

This core of knowledge of what and how to eat, is what needs to be learned and practiced over and over again to effect a lasting change. After all, what is magic but the precise performance of prescribed actions followed by specific outcomes: the MAGIC of your own HAND for weight control.

Wave your wand!

Go to PRACTICE A2 now.

Good

• Point 3

The body good goal

Who wouldn't want a quick simple solution to getting a great body? While you may hear promises that you can achieve great results with one pill or just by overloading on one food, the acquisition of good health and a great body remains omnidimensional. Nevertheless the way to **good** health and **good** muscle tone requires no special apparatus or obscure remedy. But notice I didn't say **excellent.** I'll make one assumption about you and that is that you are not seeking an Olympic gold medal. If you are, then I suggest you stop right here. But if you are not about to compete in some fitness arena, then this is what you must know. With (I'm guessing) about half the effort that it would take to become an excellent athlete you could become instead a person with a "good" level of fitness. Would you be willing to settle for good over excellent?

For your health and weight control you don't have to overdo it! The goal of **good** fitness can be easily incorporated into your present life pattern and the pursuit enjoyed.

Feeling good

The body works like a perpetual motion machine and seeks habitual patterns. If the machine is set on the "active" knob the body moves in that mode. If the machine is set on the "sedentary" knob the body literally sits in that mode. So, if you sit in an office all day, you are much more likely to continue sitting when you get home-- perhaps in front of a television set! To put it bluntly: if you're a slug, your natural tendency it to remain a slug. But, if you're a racehorse, your natural tendency is to keep running.

Changing yourself from a slug into a racehorse requires motivation. But once you make that transformation you will want to stay there. You will look great, feel better and enjoy your new world.

Moderation, however, is still the key. Body damage can occur when we push ourselves too fast, too soon. Ultimately you are the only one who knows what pace is a healthy pace for yourself on the road to physical fitness and the body good goal. Generally regular exercise of some sort every other day or about three times a week is all you will need to keep your muscles and breathing apparatus in good shape. All you really need to do is to add and maintain enough exercise to firm your body and keep it fit. The problem is often not so much what to do but how to integrate regular exercise into your daily living.

Physical fitness can be easy to acquire and maintain if the routine suits **you** and makes **you** feel great.

Adding movement

Physical activity benefits every cell in the human body. Muscle cells especially respond to movement. The heart beats faster (pumping more oxygen), the lungs expand (providing more oxygen) and the blood vessels expand (delivering more oxygen) to all the working cells of our body.

With an increase of muscle cells comes an increase of muscle tissue, and an added benefit-- an increased metabolic rate which helps to burn off calories even when you are at rest. The more muscle tissue you have, the more calorie-burning enzymes you will have at work. For these reasons physical activity is an important and necessary part of any total health and weight control program. To repeat the more muscle and less fat you have, the more energy your body will use--even at rest. This is why men tend to have a higher metabolic rate than women-- they have more muscle to begin with. The longer and more intensely you exercise, the greater the temporary boost in metabolic rate-- basically you are working harder.

Extreme dieting that results in the loss of muscle tissue is therefore counterproductive. What you want to do is lose fat tissue and gain muscle tissue. The best way for the fat person to lose weight is through a slow, but constant weight loss regimen accompanied by moderate physical activity. When you get to the last ten pounds over your ideal weight, then gradually increase the intensity of your physical activity to a level that feels comfortable and that is possible to maintain for the rest of your life.

Physical activity should be used to tone the muscles, not to lose weight. As a matter of fact, muscle tissue weighs more than fat tissue so you could actually get slimmer or firmer and gain weight! (That's why I think it's important to keep a dress or pants size in mind as well as an ideal weight.) If the scale goes up but your clothes look better then you can safely assume you're gaining muscle tissue and not fat.

The last ten pounds

If you are within the last ten pounds of your ideal weight, congratulations! But this is now when the going gets tough and the tough get going. Literally. It's time to "up" the exercise. Engage in any moderate physical activity that pleases you. My objective is only to make this health program as easy as possible for you. And once you are within ten pounds of your goal weight, the lighter weight will bring relief to all your joints, giving you more energy and ability to spring your body into shape.

If you are not within the last ten pounds of your goal weight, start easy, perhaps by toning and firming muscles. It is essential that you become aware of your body. Correct posture and correct body alignment are basic to success in almost any athletic undertaking. Many people start to run before they can walk straight! Have you ever seen someone huffing and puffing with his or her toes pointed outwards? This is asking for trouble and injury if your body is not aligned properly and one foot does not follow the other!

The pelvic tilt

When we made our evolutionary transition from four legs to two legs, we were left with a weak spot-- the lower back and abdominal muscles. Unless we make a conscientious effort to strengthen these muscles, our bellies will bulge and our backs will weaken with any physical stress. Before you engage in **any** physical activity strengthen that pelvic girdle. When you look at yourself sideways in the mirror, do you notice that your abdomen protrudes? If so it could be the result of weakened abdominal muscles as well as some excess flab. Acquiring a strong pelvic girdle will give you almost immediate results-- results that you can see in the mirror.

Now place yourself sideways in front of a good size mirror. Stand straight and see if you can pull in those abdominal muscles and tighten your buttocks. (Get up from that chair NOW.) Squeeze those buttocks as if you were holding a 50-cent piece between your cheeks. Now lie down on the floor, on your back. Follow these instructions from Ron Fletcher, author of "Every Body is Beautiful":

Lie on your back with your legs slightly parted. Ground yourself. Think of a closely dotted line from the back of your head down to your tail bone and concentrate o making each dot touch the floor. Spread your fingers over your hips, thumbs toward your pelvic bone, elbows resting on the floor. Let your legs and feet relax and turn out naturally. Now take the next five steps one at a time, slowly, precisely, and put your mind where the action is:

1. Squeeze your butt muscles.
2. Pull in your belly muscles
3. Press your lower spine into the floor.
4. Hold the position for a slow count of five.
5. Release all the muscles.
Squeeze your butt. Pull in your belly. Press your spine down.

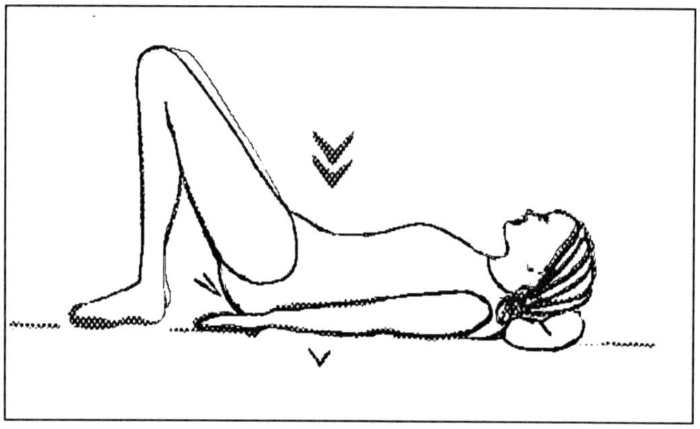

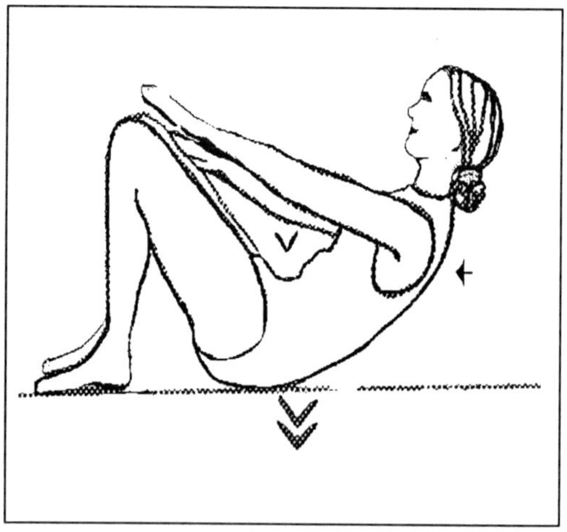

Coordinate your breathing as you tighten and release your pelvic muscles. Always **exhale as you draw in your lower abdomen** and simultaneously tighten the buttocks muscles, flattening your lower back. **Inhale when the muscles are relaxed.** In general, whenever engaging in any exercise, always remember that you should be exhaling when the muscles are tightened or contracted and that you inhale during the preceding interval when the muscles are relaxed or extended. Relax and breathe in, tighten the pelvic girdle as you breathe out. This is called abdominal breathing. (If you are inflating your chest and moving your shoulders you are not breathing properly.)

You can practice tightening the pelvic girdle almost anytime, anywhere, any time of day. Perhaps you can lie on the floor while watching television. Whether walking or bending or picking up objects from the floor, remember to keep a tight pelvic girdle, keep your spine straight, and bend your knees. You will reduce your chance of back injury and look slimmer even if you don't lose a pound. Women especially should avoid high-heeled shoes, that is, any shoe with a heel higher than two inches. Check your sleeping position-- a rounded back is best, sleeping on the side with a bend to the knees. Whenever you get the opportunity, tilt that pelvis and tighten those buttocks. Eventually, without thinking, your body will retain the strengthened position. Avoid letting it all hang out!

You can also stand against a wall and get similar benefit by pressing your back against the wall, closing the hollow part of your back. Try this. With the heels of your feet no more than a foot away from the wall, pull in your abdominal muscles and flatten your back against the wall. If you are doing this exercise correctly, your hand will not fit between your back and the wall surface. This is a great exercise to do while waiting for elevators, or, in fact, waiting any place where you can find a flat wall. I often do my pelvic tilt while I am walking or while I am standing in line at the supermarket or at a sales counter. (I use the time!) One woman told me that she does her pelvic tilts while housecleaning. Every time she walks through a doorway, she stops and tilts! As a result, she looks terrific with a firm and flat "stomach". Become conscious of your mid-area and select the situation or routine that suits you.

Some foot-rules

I know that you think you know how to walk. After all, just like breathing, you've been walking just fine. So, let's take the tell-tale test. Find any pair of flat-soled shoes (loafers, tennis shoes, or sandals, etc.). Look at the bottom of your shoes. If either edge of the heel is worn down, it means that you are not walking properly. The wear on your shoe should be fairly even from the edge of the inner heel around to the big toe. Stand about five steps away from your full-length mirror again and watch yourself walk. Walk towards the mirror. Do your feet turn outward or are the toes marching straight ahead? Here's a description of what should happen from Charles T. Kuntzleman's "The Complete Book of Walking":

Each foot should strike the ground at your heel. The weight is then transferred from your heel up along the outer border of your foot toward your toes. Then you should push off with your toes to complete the foot strike pattern. As you move from heel to toe, you will get a rolling motion. Avoid landing flat footed and on the balls of your feet.

A prerequisite to any strenuous physical activity is mastering the pelvic tilt and a straight walk. Put your body in line before you play.

Keep your head erect, toes straight forward and arms swinging as they brush against your side. As the left foot advances, the right arm swings forward, and as your right foot advances, the left arm swings forward. And remember to keep that pelvic girdle tight. Walking is perhaps the most natural physical activity for us now erect two-legged Homo sapiens. Almost everybody walks and I hope you'll be walking for the rest of your life-- so do it right. Stand straight, keep the body relaxed but erect, throw back your shoulders, pull in your abdomen and buttocks and walk straight. Do **all this** with a smile on your face!

Stepping high

The main reasons for moving your body are to bring oxygen to the cells through more rapid and deeper breathing, to exercise the muscles beyond normal use, and to gain an awareness of your physical being. When we were children we played in the streets, in our backyards and in playgrounds, joyfully laughing romping, running and teasing. We had fun! Let us bring back the physical play we once knew in childhood. Exercise need not be a chore. When we exercise simply to lose weight or to satisfy someone else's demands (like a gym teacher's), what was once fun becomes work. Forget about the benefits of exercise and concentrate on the joy it can bring. Think about it. What did you really enjoy as a youngster? Was it skipping rope? Shooting hoops?

The best exercise for you is the one you'll do consistently and enjoy. I could present a large table describing the benefit of each sport, but I do not believe that any one exercise should be selected over others because of superiority in a selected factor. Physical activity, of almost any kind, will increase your awareness of your body and build your muscle tissue. Do not concern yourself with whether an activity is considered aerobic (without oxygen debt) or anaerobic (with oxygen debt). Obviously, you can sustain an activity for a longer length of time without stopping if you don't run out of oxygen! Many sports combine both qualities. For example, although swimming is considered an aerobic activity, occasionally the swimmer will experience an oxygen debt, improving his or her overall aerobic capability.

What's important is that you get out and move. Or stay inside, and move. Truly the best exercise in the one you enjoy doing the most.

And flexibility is important for either aerobic or anaerobic exercises. So, do not choose an activity because it is either aerobic or anaerobic or promotes flexibility. Keep in mind that some people are better suited for one type of exercise than another. For example, if you lack flexibility, you may be more prone to injury if you take up jogging. If you are flexible, the balance beam or yoga or ballet my come easily to you. Some of us are tight-jointed and some of us are loose-jointed. Also, some of us have more sprint fiber than endurance fiber.

But maybe it's been so long that you no longer remember what you used to enjoy doing. It might be helpful to know something about your body type and what sports might come more easily to you than others. Maybe you can tell what abilities you have by identifying the sports that are easy for you.

Explosive ability

Sports demanding this athletic trait are tennis, squash, football, water-skiing, boxing and racquetball. In many of these sports you may experience an oxygen deficit, making them anaerobic type exercises.

Endurance ability

These sports develop lung capacity. Sports requiring endurance ability are cross-country skiing, cycling, mountaineering, crew, skating, aerobic dancing and speed roller skating. You will get the aerobic benefit as long as you can still "talk" while moving.

Flexibility

Put your left hand behind your back. Point your fingers toward your shoulder blades. Now, put your right hand over your right shoulder and try to touch your fingers. If your fingers touch or cross, you are flexible.

Skiing, figure-skating, wind-surfing, gymnastics, yoga and ballet all require flexibility.

Selecting physical play

Our body type, muscle strength, muscle endurance and flexibility may make the difference in our enjoyment of a selected sport. However, just because it's easier for you to do one thing over another is not a reason in itself to pursue the sport. You might enjoy selecting a sport that increases your flexibility if you're not flexible or increases your lung capacity if you have low endurance. Just as there is no one magic food that will bring you wellness, there is also no one magic sport that will bring you all encompassing physical fitness.

Your physical play must meet several requirements-- it must be fun, it must be something you can do without too much strain, and in short, it must be play. Your physical play time perhaps could bring back some good childhood memories. It could also introduce you to a new sport and new people.

Think back to all the wonderful playtimes you had as a child. When you went outdoors to play, wasn't it fun? Did you play hopscotch, or jump rope, or run up and down the block playing hide and seek? When it snowed did you go sledding? And when it rained did you have fun sloshing around in your boots? Or, did you stay inside and dance to records? When summer came, were you anxious to get to the beach? Did you have fun building sand castles and jumping the big waves? What **were** your fun play activities in childhood?

I encourage you to get out there and do what seems like fun. If it makes you laugh while you're trying to do the Charleston, or it makes you laugh when you miss a badminton birdie so much the better for your effort.

Part of the fun of learning a new sport is not being able to do everything perfectly. Keep your sense of humor and compete only with yourself. All that matters is that **you're** having a good time while others are sitting home watching television.

All you really need is to find one sport that you find appealing. With time you may want to explore others. Variety, however, **is** the spice of life and the more sports that you enjoy, the greater will be your choice of activity and the less likely you are to become bored. You can become mediocre in a large number of sports and still enjoy them!

Plan for the season and select some form of physical play that is the most convenient and easy for you to implement in your daily life. Many activities are only enjoyable if the weather is good. I won't tell you to go jogging in the rain unless it is something you genuinely find fun. The season, the weather, the equipment needed and convenience of the activity are all important factors contributing to the desirability of any sport. Convenience and joy are the ingredients necessary to make a regular physical activity program feasible.

Consider your present situation. Do you live in the country or the city? I've discovered that walking out my front door requires very little motivation, and getting into a car and lugging equipment requires more effort and can make the difference between my getting some physical play or not. When I lived in New York City I was able to make use of an indoor swimming pool located between my office and my residence. I would stop en route on the subway, get off for a swim; then I would get back on the subway and continue home. When I lived in San Francisco, swimming was out of the question. The only pools were indoor pools inconveniently located, so I walked. But, when I lived in Escondido, I had a swimming pool and tennis courts across the street at a country club where I had membership. When I lived in La Jolla, there was a pool in my building complex. When I lived in Del Mar I walked the hills of my neighborhood. And living in Seal Beach I have a pool in my backyard! In New York City swimming was "on my way home" and now in Seal Beach literally outside my door.

Ideally any activity played outside your home or located somewhere between your office and home or within a ten minute walk from your home or office is the one to pick. Convenience does contribute to regularity, but if your favorite activity isn't outside your front door, judge for yourself if the travel time or distance is a negative factor.

Some of the health clubs are so attractive they just might be worth the extra effort it takes to get in the car and go. And some activities are so much fun, these seemingly minor considerations are of little consequence. Know yourself. Select the physical play activity that **is** possible for you to do right **now--** in this season. If you need equipment or classes or a partner they can be acquired later. Right now, select an activity that would be good for you. Have you selected your physical play?

Mind over matter

Perhaps you've heard that famous athletes have used mental imagery to guide their playing on the football field or to better place tennis balls. It's true. It can work for you. Now you can start to focus on seeing yourself with your ideal body participating in the sport you just selected. If you selected dancing, imagine yourself putting on your leotards and dancing shoes, stretching and whirling to the music. Affirm that you will buy or get from your closet the necessary equipment and clothes needed for your selected sport. See yourself as this dancer (or whatever sport you chose) and increase your awareness of others who dance. When you watch television, notice the dancers. See yourself in the role. Go to the library and browse through the many books on dancing. Look for dance magazines or through other popular magazines for photos of dancers. Find a hero- someone you admire who does your sport. Think dance. Visualize yourself literally following in the footsteps of your heroine or hero. If you were previously sedentary this mental preparation will ease your transition to a physically active being.

You are getting the mental preparation to transform your self-image. You must see yourself as someone who can do this activity, whatever you selected, and see yourself as fit and trim. The action will follow. You can also just go ahead and do it, but it's an easier transition if you can see yourself in the picture first. Get ready mentally, get set with the proper equipment and you'll be champing at the bit to get out of the gate!

The right equipment

Committing yourself to any physical activity means acquiring the equipment needed to safely and efficiently participate in the sport. You'll need good walking shoes if you're going to walk. You'll need perhaps a sunhat and goggles, bathing suit, and lessons if you're going to swim. Don't forget good shoes, shorts and shirt and a well-strung racket and balls that bounce if you're going to play tennis. Without the right equipment you reduce your potential for joy in sport and encourage defeat. Educate yourself on your selected physical play. Even if you think you know how to ride a bike or do yoga handstands or lift weights, read the beginner books. You may pick up a few pointers, but more importantly, the written word will motivate you to act. When I decided to start swimming again, I was shocked to learn that I didn't know **how** to swim. I'd been swimming off and on for years. I took some elementary lessons and discovered how little I really knew. Techniques had changed and there were new theories on how to place your arms. As a result, I am confident now that I am swimming to the best of my ability although I guarantee there are no Olympic medals in sight. I am a slug in the water! But, I love the sport. However, I did improve my stroke and I now swim by alternating my head from side to side as I breathe which I discovered helped me to relax more. Read about your sport. Get the proper equipment. And take lessons or a refresher course if necessary.

A contingency plan

O.K. So what happens when you're all set to go for that great game of tennis and the heavens open with an unexpected downpour? What happens when a blizzard appears on the slopes or your square dance partner doesn't show up? We can become easily thwarted in our new physical play program by a change in weather or a change in circumstances if we do not have a good **alternative**. It's a back-up, a last resort, a way to maintain your physical fitness if all else fails.

Review your list of enjoyable activities and discover which ones might be suitable for indoors or as a back-up. Again, be prepared. When the weather is bad, use your contingency plan. When you are traveling, use your contingency plan. Do not limit yourself to one sport-- use changes in weather and changes in circumstances as opportunities to explore other activities. You can watch television while riding a stationery bicycle. Or, you may find a television program on yoga or aerobic dancing which you can follow at home. Or perhaps you can insert a moderately programmed workout video into a player and follow along. There **are** alternatives. You can develop your own indoor exercise program (to music!) by grouping together specific exercises designed to strengthen and tone your physical problem areas. Most people need to strengthen their abdominals, buttocks and the back of the arms to look and feel good. Find the spot exercises that will do that for you and make them part of your contingency plan-- an indoor exercise you can do on a rainy day. Just pick the spot exercises that feel right to you, are not too challenging, and seem to do some good. If you have a contingency plan, an alternative to your selected sports, neither hail, nor rain, nor sleet, nor snow will keep you from your physical play period.

A continuous performance

Use it or lose it. When it comes to the body that is the message we get. In order to physiologically benefit from physical play, it must be practiced regularly. More important than the specific sport you have chosen or the intensity of the activity, is the regularity with which it is pursued. Fortunately, one need not exercise every day in order to maintain a good level of fitness. Having this leeway makes it possible for us to juggle our schedules. Certainly, you can afford 20 minutes of physical play three times a week. That's all you need. The truth is, you can't afford **not** to exercise.

Adding movement to your life contributes to reversing bodily degeneration and reducing risk factors associated with many chronic diseases. If you **don't** move, the body suffers gradual deterioration-- called hypokinetic disease. Need I say more? Almost all researchers agree that in order to maintain a good level of physical conditioning, one should exercise regularly. However, giving your body a rest between physical play periods allows the body to dissipate accumulated fatigue products associated with increased blood pressure and cardiac output. How often should you exercise? How long?

The guidelines have now relaxed from what they were years ago. Fitness experts used to recommend strenuous physical activity for at least 20 minutes at least three times a week. I still think it's a good idea. But, if you can't accomplish that feat, take heart. More moderate exercise done over the course of the day can also keep you healthy. Walking to work, climbing stairs, cleaning your car, or gardening can meet similar health goals as long as these activities add up to at least 30 minutes a day. For example, you could take a 10 minute walk on your way to work, climb stairs over the course of the day for a total of 10 minutes, and then wash your car vigorously for 10 minutes when you come home. It would be best to structure these activities into your daily routine, so that they will become habitual. Link them to your work break or to something that will generally stay in place. Keep in mind the joy factor. If adding movement during the course of your day simply becomes another chore rethink your activities. Would it be fun to park your car at the end of the lot so that you will automatically walk farther? Would it be fun to walk to a store rather than drive?

Here is the rule: Every other day exercise to accumulate 30 minutes or exercise for a continuous 20 minutes.

Do what is easiest for you and what you would enjoy the most. It is a matter of planning an exercise routine that fits your lifestyle so that it meets the criterion of either an accumulated 30 minutes over the course of the day; or a steady 20-30 minutes of physical play during the day.

Whatever type of exercise you select or routine you follow, the training effect will not last unless your activity is continued at regular intervals. More frequent, but less intensive bouts of activity are actually better for you than less frequent, more intensive bouts of physical exertion. Take the slow, paced approach, but in order not to lose the training effect, never allow more than two days to pass without some physical activity.

Our goal is to establish an enjoyable activity that you can incorporate into your present life at regular intervals. If you decide to accumulate minutes, I suggest (to keep track of your accumulated 30 minutes of exercise) that you use your left hand to count minutes! Make each finger represent five minutes. Then when you run out of fingers, the last five minutes is in the "V" for victory between your thumb and index finger to signify that you've met the 30 minute criterion.

Body wisdom

The duration of your physical play period will vary according to the type of exercise you have chosen and your physical condition.

To gain physiological results, in all sports, the objective is to get more oxygen into your lungs and to move your muscles beyond normal use. It has been said that you must never exercise to get in shape, but that you must be in shape to exercise. You must know yourself and judge whether a physical activity is bringing you, not only pleasure, but results-- more vigorous breathing and muscle power. Even bowling and sailing can be useful activities if you are continuously moving, remembering to breathe deeply and stretching at every opportunity. Obviously, some activities are more rigorous than others. Does your physical activity increase your pulse rate, deepen your breathing and work your muscles? After all, if you walk in slow motion or ride in a golf cart, you'll get no physical benefit. So, when you garden, garden with vigor. And if you decide that washing your car is what you enjoy, do it at a brisk pace-- enough to raise your pulse and work your muscles. Almost any activity can become a conditioning activity if you keep these principles in mind. The more intensive the exercise, however, the less time you will need to obtain a conditioning benefit. You must become tuned to your body and know when enough is enough. Your body is sending messages to you all the time. If you listen you will acquire body sense.

Become conscious of your body's limitations. Never pull or strain a muscle until it hurts. Pain is a sign of fatigue and a signal that you should stop. Gradually build up your muscle strength, only slightly stressing yourself. And always, when you are engaging in aerobic activities, be sure that you are breathing comfortably enough to pass the "talk" test-- meaning that you are able to carry on a conversation while participating in the sport. If you feel exceptionally tired or fatigued after physical play, you probably overdid it. Don't' fall into the trap of over-exertion-- that's how to become a quitter. Remember what you are seeking-- a physiological response to a small amount of exercise. I assume that you are not aspiring to become a professional athlete. They work hard and sometimes very strenuously to maintain a competitive edge. Work into your program gradually and slowly.

Moderation is the key. Learn to recognize the warning signals of over-exertion. If your heart is racing and your breath is short-- stop. Slow down to a comfortable pace, even if it is a slow shuffle. Getting your body into shape is only a matter of training, and you can do it at your own pace.

Use your body wisdom. And don't worry about what others may think. Occasionally I will be outdone during my fast-walk by a jogger or runner or another fast-walker. My natural reaction is, "I'm not doing enough. She (or He)'s much better than I am." Not so. You are doing what is right for you and hopefully the speedy person that passed you by isn't straining his or her muscles and is at the right pace for himself. When I swim laps in the pool, the same thing happens. Inevitably someone else will start to do laps with greater vigor than I, and I start to feel inferior, but then I remind myself that my pace is the right pace for me. Don't listen to well-meaning friends, your wife or husband, or athletes. Listen only to your body.

Tapping your toes

You will discover that some of the physical play activities you enjoy are more demanding than others. For cardiovascular conditioning, the four "best exercises" are bicycling, walking, jogging and swimming. Of these, women are especially well suited for swimming because of their extra layer of fat giving them natural buoyancy. Because of a woman' wider pelvis, she is more prone to injuries in the lower part of the body--

legs, ankles, feet and knees. In general, for both men and women, I recommend avoiding activities with an excess of bouncing or compression severe enough to damage body tissues. Joggers land heel first and the heel withstands a force equal to 150 percent of the body's weight. If you are overweight, this is why you are at high risk for knee and foot injuries. Short men with a flexible and light body type do well as joggers, but tall men may be asking for trouble.

Your energy level, present physical condition and personal idiosyncrasies will determine the physical play activities best suited for yourself at this time. You must learn to recognize what sports are "good" for you. If the activity doesn't feel good or if you don't like it, don't do it. The crucial element is to find pleasure in the activity. Avoid the extremes, become conscious of your body type, gauge your energy level, and your body will stay in tune.

The transition from a sedentary life-style to an active one is often difficult and it is for this reason that we have spent so much time warming up to the idea. I have given you the secrets to success. If you know that you are a person who can dive into a fitness program and stay with it-- more power to you! If, on the other hand, you have already made several attempts at the fitness game and are no longer participating in any physical activity, then I suggest you follow all of these recommendations:

1. Start to strengthen your body in preparation for physical play. Become conscious of your pelvic girdle and strengthen your abdominal and low back muscles.

2. Maintain your pelvic belt consciousness and practice walking with your body in correct alignment. Check the heels of your shoes and see that your feet do not "toe in" or "toe out". Your feet should follow a straight line.

3. Visualize yourself participating in physical play. Mentally imagine yourself engaging in your favorite activity.

4. Develop a contingency plan for alternate physical play activities if the weather or circumstances change, not permitting you your regular activity.

5. Find times during the day when it is convenient for you to have physical play. If you choose a 20 minute session, I recommend playing about one hour before a meal or 2 hours after a meal.

6. If, once started in physical play, you no longer enjoy the activity after one or two tries, quit! Find another play activity that feels like fun.

7. Be sure to have the proper equipment appropriate for your physical play activity. Read books on your sport for pointers or take lessons from an expert who will not push you too quickly.

8. Start your physical play program slowly. Plan to play once a week at first, and then graduate to twice a week and so on until you reach the physical play guidelines every other day.

9. Remember this important rule: Every other day exercise for an accumulated 30 minutes or exercise for a continuous 20 minute session.

Establish the **regularity** of your physical play program before you establish the intensity. Because change is stressful introduce each change slowly. Take it one step at a time.

Any exercise is better than no exercise!

Go to PRACTICE G3 now.

*I*nner

● Point 4

How do I eat every day?

In this Point we will discuss what is "food" for the soul, for that part of us that screams to be filled. And for that part of us that feels empty. It is not enough to know what to do to effect weight loss. You have the facts. You have the knowledge. But there are other factors that need to be addressed to insure your success. Truly the easy part is learning how to eat properly. The difficulty so many of us face is controlling the demons within that may sabotage our best efforts. The need for other's approval is often very strong and the wrong reason for losing weight. Without nurturing the part of us that needs attention, love, and caring our efforts to lose weight are futile. How we eat, our personal style of consumption, is often related more to psychological factors than the physical hunger we believe we are satisfying.

May I ask, "How do you eat?" On the surface this may seem like an odd question, but the answer may reveal why one is having a problem with being overweight. Whatever you are presently eating and whatever style or pattern you have adopted for meals and snacks represents the weight-gain diet you're already on. It's nonsense to say diets don't work because they do-- either for you or against you. People are always telling me that they hate diets and they refuse to go on a diet. What we must realize is that we are already on a diet of our own making. It is "Ellen's put on 10 pounds in three months diet". Or it is "Jack's gain 6 pounds in one meal program". A diet simply is what you usually eat and drink-- your daily fare. A diet is not a two-week quick fix. We tend to view diets as temporary and negative because they are associated with short-term deprivation. The diet you are already on is what you generally eat, in the quantities you are used to eating. If you are now overweight, your normal diet is probably a weight-gain diet and **that** is what we will modify into a weight loss and maintenance diet.

Some people are lucky and just naturally seem to know when to stop eating and like the foods that help them to maintain good health. These people either learned at an early age how to eat and it's "natural" to them, or by nature were endowed with good genes, a high metabolic rate, and sense. Most of us who are overweight just lack inner controls. We really don't know how to eat properly to maintain our health and ideal body weight. And in many cases our genes are not on our side and our natural physiology is set to accumulate fat, so, according to biological theory, we can ride out periods of starvation in icy blizzards. We who collect fat were good survivors in the Stone Age. But times have changed. We really don't need to store that much energy anymore and we've become long-lived people. We also know a lot more. We know that living longer and being healthy, feeling good and physically able are all associated with being trim.

Our style of eating has changed too. When we were hunter-gatherers we might have always been a little hungry waiting for the next meal. There were times of feast and famine. In most cities food is available 24 hours a day. We live in a time of constant feast. Only those who are economically deprived face the fear of famine. Ironically, the rich in the United States strive to be thin while the poor often console themselves with food. Our relationship to food in this age many times is socially based.

We have "breakfast meetings", we "do lunch" and we "invite to dinner". Based on physiology and our blood-sugar levels, spacing these meals about 4 hours apart seems to make good sense. The structure of our eating day tends to follow our natural biology and blood sugar levels.

I have classified the types and styles of unhealthy eating into three major categories: High Intake Appestat (HIA), Trigger Food Bingeing (TFB), and Stuffing Feelings Eating (SFE). (And of course, there is a healthy type of eating, Healthy Balanced Eating--HBE-- the style of eating that will not lead to weight gain.) If you are an overweight person reading this book most likely your style of eating is represented by one of the three unhealthy eating type classifications.

High intake appestat

HIA (**H**igh **I**ntake **A**ppestat) eaters are those people who simply do not know when to stop eating. Their physical "appestat" is in the wrong gear. They need to readjust their brains (literally) to give a stop signal at another level. These people gain weight because they just eat too much! Or, put another way, they do not know when to stop. They are the easiest to cure, and sometimes they don't need to change their diet at all. Especially for men, regular exercise can go a long way towards curbing extra weight.

Trigger food bingeing

TFB (**T**rigger **F**ood **B**ingeing) involves a complicated mix of wrong signals to the brain and psychological dysfunction. Anyone who suffers from bingeing knows that they become out of control. The trigger to a binge episode can sometimes be a certain food or a pressure exerted on a psychological button. This eater may eat until feeling nauseous or sick, but will still want to eat more. If you are a trigger food binger, you know that you just can't stop eating once you start to indulge in some specific food (like a potato chip or cookie).

Some TFB's are also "Stuffing Feelings Eaters" (SFE's), stuffing their feelings trying fill their "hole in the soul", often not facing their anger. In essence the trigger here is a situation.

Stuffing feelings eating

Not all SFE's are necessarily binge eaters. Stuffing your feelings could be a chronic situation where certain foods are selected to make yourself feel good when what you are actually feeling is too disturbing or painful to acknowledge. A true SFE (**S**tuffing **F**eelings **E**ating) person has episodic bouts of eating for pleasure, perhaps going through an entire pint of ice cream at one sitting when feeling low or the next day eating an entire bag of potato chips to enjoy watching a football game. The SFE person is not totally out of control. However, this type of eating is most significantly "problem eating" since ill health consequences may result from being overweight or over-eating. If the physical results of your over-eating mean that you require medical attention (high blood pressure, heart disease), then you are very likely this type of eater.

Learning how to eat will help the binge eater to gain some control over eating. A deprivation diet would be the worst diet for a binger, since as soon as it's over and before it begins two irresistible opportunities for bingeing will have presented themselves. Generally, the binger already feels deprived, so a deprivation diet just exacerbates this dysfunctional type of eating behavior. It is important for the binger to come to terms with his or her feelings if stuffing feelings or to recognize that certain foods are physiological triggers.

Psychological counseling is often beneficial. On your own you can document your bingeing episodes, write down your feelings, the time and date of occurrence and the food chosen. You may see a consistent pattern and understand your own behavior better. Ask yourself what you are trying to "fill"? Also ask what you are accomplishing by bingeing. Sabotage? Proving to yourself that you're not good? What? With concentrated self-exploration and the guidance of a professional counselor, you may be able to get at the root of the problem.

Many of us are all three types, High Intake Appestat, Trigger Food Binger, and Stuffing Feelings Eater at different times. Try to determine what type of eating you think is most responsible for your weight gains? Are you simply a Thanksgiving and Christmas overeater who gains five to eight pounds every year? Or can you not be in the same room with a bag of peanuts without devouring them totally and looking for more? Or are you chronically trying to make yourself feel good by overindulging with treats?

Mind control

You already know how to eat because you have learned *MAGIC-HAND* eating. But you will sabotage yourself over and over again if you do not understand the psychological underpinnings causing your overeating in the first place. So, let's look at all three types of eating to determine what must be done to gain the mind control you need to be successful.

<u>High Intake Appestat:</u>

Your problem basically is that you just eat too much, probably on "special" occasions and in general whenever food is put on the table. Food may be your ""lover", too. You enjoy the company of this food so much that a little more or an extra helping fills a small hole somewhere that says I need love. (Or, I need a friend.)

Many brain chemicals affect hunger and knowing when to stop eating is a message that must get to the brain. Our appetite center is located in the hypothalamus, near the base of brain. Specialized nerve cells monitor glucose levels in the blood signaling our feelings of hunger. Some people take longer than others to turn off the hunger signal or have a delayed reaction to the feeling of being "satiated" and will overeat on a regular basis.

People with a High Intake Appestat will generally have an extra two or three servings at a meal when others around them have stopped at one serving. Are you someone who always has an extra serving when asked because you don't feel filled yet?

Trigger Food Bingeing:

Your problem is that certain foods trigger a physiological response that becomes almost uncontrollable for more of the same. In other arenas of your life you may also be an obsessive-compulsive personality. In some people, the physiological craving for sugar starts a snowball response to all sweetened foods. Ice cream and chocolate bars are the two foods people most frequently crave. Sugar and starchy foods generally have a calming effect. Research shows that carbohydrates release the brain chemical serotonin, which is believed to reduce feelings of anxiety and frustration. Serotonin uses tryptophan as its chemical source which is obtained in the diet from poultry, fish, lean meat and peanuts. But these foods must be balanced in the diet with a carbohydrate (like pasta) in order for the serotonin to make it to the brain.

Specific foods, commonly sugar and alcohol, react with chemicals in the brain and can set us up for depression or anxiety after a temporary high. In addition, people may have allergies to such foods as eggs, wheat, soybeans, citrus fruit and milk.

In essence we are all unique chemistry sets. And it is quite possibly true that "one man's meat is another man's poison". L-phenylalanine is the amino acid that converts into two neurotransmitters: norepinephrine and dopamine. The desire for food, not actual hunger, may be a way to appease a temporary negative emotional upheaval. Emotional triggers linked to binge eating can become addictive similar to the type of behavior exhibited by an alcoholic who "can't stop". A conscious and focused effort will be required to control the abuse of (anesthetizing "feel better") food as a solution to psychological disruptions.

Eating becomes addictive because it feels good and physiologically you are triggering endorphins. So when you are feeling down, you may be seeking an upper. The "upper" could be a food that triggers the release of endorphins in the brain, that once started becomes an obsessive demand.

Stuffing Feelings Eating:

Your problem is that you get comfort from food. Food may spell love. So, how can you make yourself feel better without resorting to food? Research suggests that three days of bad moods out of ten days is average and that the hardest mood to shake is anger. However, what most people fail to realize is that it is possible to exert control over their moods. I know that when you're so far down it's hard to get up.

The most effective way to lift a depression is to take some **action**--just do something no matter how trivial to solve the problem that is creating your bad mood. (But, don't eat!) If you need some oral "comfort-gratification" make yourself some hot tea or find another low or no-calorie drink that soothes you and drink it through a straw. (How about coffee with a touch of Hershey's cocoa and some milk or cinnamon to satisfy the love means chocolate need?) A long walk might be the best antidote for anger and this makes sense to me. Remember that when we're angry our adrenaline rises demanding physical expression. A walk might be just as good as punching someone out.

It might be helpful if you can identify your feelings and know if you are angry or depressed. Remember that depression often follows unexpressed anger. So if you **are** depressed, what are you angry about? The chances are good that what we really are stuffing is our anger. Anger usually comes from a threat, a loss, and/or hurt. We can become threatened when someone violates our personal space in some way. For example, if someone continuously stepped on your toes either physically or psychologically, you'd get angry. Loss can occur in many situations. We can think we have failed in some way, we could lose a possession or an ability, or a loved one, and we could lose a part of our life that was important to our identity. Whenever we lose something of value, we might feel depressed. The simple answer is to seek love from another source, not from food. May I suggest attending a religious service or listening to a singing group or choir? You might feel "filled" instead with spiritual love. Being in harmony with others whether in a singing group or on a dance floor can fill some empty spaces.

The "need" to eat may be traced to a violation of your physical or emotional boundaries either presently or from the past. You may be eating to add protection-- to put a fence of fat so to speak to protect from further violation. Many overly "sensitive" people are actually people with loose boundaries. Their sense of self may be very open and vulnerable to assault from the outside because their psychological defenses were poorly developed as a result of repeated childhood trauma.

Perhaps you can identify some "lost love". Food may be numbing the feeling of the pain of that loss. Food is a lover and eating is a way of coping. Extra layers of fat offer "protection". As one lonely overweight teenager stated, "Look at me. You can see that food is my best friend." Ask yourself, "Am I trying to fill some "emptiness" with food?"

You may see yourself as a victim; you may feel discounted or ignored and powerless. Whatever may have happened to you has much to do with how you have interpreted the situation. The psychological part of problem eating is the inability to express the emotions you are feeling. In therapy the emotional aspect can often be resolved in relation to the event. For someone else a similar event may not have left an open wound. Your healing and the approach you take is a very personal matter.

The chronically angry person usually feels powerless in their present situation, but in fact may have more control than they think. Our feelings of powerlessness often stem from our childhoods even though as adults we are now more in control. Behind most of our anger is a deep hurt, and if it is intense enough, you may need to seek professional counseling. Dealing with your hurts, healing the wounds, should go a long way towards alleviating the need to stuff yourself with food to avoid the pain of feeling what you don't want to feel. In short, you must learn to stop *feeding* your *feelings*.

To summarize, we eat for many reasons. Most emotional eating is fear-based. The threat of hurt or loss causes us to feel anxious so we may eat to "protect" ourselves. After we get hurt, we may become angry and we eat to stuff the feeling. If the anger is unresolved, we may become depressed. If we are lonely because of lost love we may feel sorry for ourselves, and we eat for comfort, or to feel better.

Mood chemistry

Nutrients do appear to impact brain neurotransmitters. As you may recall from high school biology, a neuron is a brain cell. Tiny electrical impulses travel from one neuron to another via brain chemicals and these chemical highways are called neurotransmitters. Your brain chemistry is influenced by what you eat, how you exercise, your interactions with other people and your environment. You thoughts and feelings are greatly influenced by the chemistry of your brain.

When brain chemicals fluctuate you are likely to experience wide changes in mood. Most women are keenly aware of how their normally sunny disposition can change during a pre-menstrual fluctuation of estrogen and progesterone hormone levels. Although less recognized, men too have similar hormonal mood swings. In general, everyone is subject to thought and mood swings as a result of his or her biochemistry.

Cravings

The brain not only turns your appetite on and off, it also may make you hungrier for specific foods. A blood sample can determine if you have the fat gene responsible for "sugar craving". This gene is also linked to alcohol and drug addiction. In essence the brain is a chemical organ and sugars increase the amount of the neurotransmitters giving pleasurable feelings. Your physical and psychological environment will determine to what extent food, alcohol or drugs will be used to stimulate this pleasure center. To get off any substance addiction it is necessary to alleviate the underlying psychological pain and/or find a healthier pleasure substitute. Maybe as the song says, all you need is love.

Many people believe that artificially flavored sugared drinks are the answer to their sweet tooth. Unfortunately, your body knows when it's being tricked, and the artificial sweetener may actually set you up for a real sugar binge. The sweet taste tricks the body into producing insulin in anticipation for calories. When the calories don't appear you may actually feel hungrier. You would be better advised to drink a naturally flavored mineral water with no artificial sweetener.

Jumping through the hoop

So, how can you feel good about yourself? For starters, think about your successes in life. See yourself as a person who is already successful because you are doing the right things for yourself (like reading this book). If there is something that you need to change or improve think of yourself as on your way to that goal. It might be helpful to cut out inspirational or "feel good" articles or sayings and put them in an album or folder to refer to whenever you need a lift. Or perhaps you have a favorite piece of music you could play.

Remember that taking some action will help to counteract bad feelings when they start to take a grip. We all face periods of self-doubt, we all wonder about ourselves, and that is human nature and part of our growth process. You must find your own truth to have inner harmony.

Taking control

A growing body of research tells us that personality may play a significant role in health. Emotions and attitude can either fortify or depress the immune system affecting the body's ability to heal itself.

Moods can also be highly contagious. If you are in a "toxic relationship" with another person you may notice that you feel "less than" or anxious or depressed after being with him or her. People who are more empathetic towards others are more likely than others to pick up the moods around them. So, help yourself and others-- put on a happy face!

Self-talk

It is important to address the subconscious needs you may have for keeping your weight. If you lose a lot of weight and then gain it back it may mean that you have an underlying fear connected with the weight loss. Your pounds may have been protecting you from something. Do you have some inner fear? Who is it that didn't love you enough? The mind will direct the body to gain weight to protect itself. Talk to yourself about your fears. Ask yourself how you can overcome the obstacle, and answer with the solution that you discover from your own self-talk. An answer from someone else may be considered, but put yourself in charge of the final decision. You can solve many of your own problems through this simple process of self-talk, which I believe most children freely engage, but adults tend to neglect.

Everyone has ups and downs in life. Think of what you can say to yourself to bring yourself "up".

The magic key

The way you behave, the way you think, and the way you feel directly influences your physical being. Ultimately **you** must make the decision to change your injurious behavioral habits and adopt new behaviors for a healthier eating lifestyle. I can give you all sorts of suggestions, and provide a blueprint, but nothing will happen until you decide to take hold of your life. You can do something about your physicality. You have the power to change yourself. You simply must decide to make it happen. Ask yourself over and over again how you can make this *MAGIC-HAND* Eating Plan your way of life, how you could make it fun for yourself, and how you could not feel deprived. When you get the solution to an obstacle, then test your answer.

Let me tell you how a little self-searching can work in a positive way. I had a terrible problem keeping track of what seemed like an unending stream of papers entering my office. (My office is in my home.) The problem was that I hated sorting through papers and it was difficult for me to take action on so many things I received in the mail. I kept putting off responses to business correspondence and social invitations and I felt bogged down. Plus, occasionally I'd lose a check! Finally one day **I decided** that I had to find a solution to this problem. Nothing I tried had worked. But I had never tried to make sorting papers fun. What could I do to make this horrible (for me) task fun? I tried to think of what would be fun. I like to dance. Was there some way I could combine the two? My answer was to set the timer on my oven for one hour and see how many papers I could clear up in that time. As I sorted papers, responded to correspondence, and located files, I would dance in-between tasks to music playing softly in the background. It felt wonderful to get things done! I now love what I call my "paper hour".

You must decide to conquer whatever could be holding you back from successful weight loss and find your own happy solutions to psychological, attitudinal or relationship obstacles. Keep asking yourself questions (What am I feeling? Can I find comfort when needed by doing something other than eating?) and you will discover the answers. Take a walk. Smell the roses. Take a bath. Talk to a friend. Be determined.

Make the **decision** to go for victory. Don't stuff. Take action.

Feel the feeling.

Go to PRACTICE I4 now.

Control

• Point 5

Time on your hands

Funny, isn't it? Who these days has any time on their hands? Most of us are oversubscribed between our work, our families and the various demands of maintaining a household. It would be funny if it wasn't so true. Somewhere in our busy schedules we must find the time to stay healthy. In fact very little time is needed to stay healthy, but to "make the time", a change in routine may be needed.

What is the actual time you will need to stay healthy? For exercise, the absolute minimum would be 1 hour a week in spaced intervals and whatever duration you prefer. This could mean 20 minutes of vigorous walking three days a week or 10 minutes of stair climbing every day but Sunday. For eating, finding time doesn't seem to be a problem unless you are preparing elaborate menus. Most of us eat regular meals and finding time places no extra burden. Using your *MAGIC-HAND*, you might need five extra minutes a day to count your finger-palm and thumb-joint portions. That's all. For your spiritual health, I recommend 20 minutes a day of quiet time, inner reflection, or meditation. This amounts to 2 hours and 20 minutes a week. To maintain your health the greatest allotment of time will go to simply sitting still! This spiritual requirement is what I feel will keep you in balance so that you have the psychological "space" to stay with your *MAGIC-HAND* Eating Plan and the energy and motivation to stay with a regular program of exercise.

All together you must find three hours and twenty-five minutes a week to devote to staying healthy. **3 HOURS AND 25 MINUTES.** So, the question is, where will you find three hours and twenty-five minutes a week in your busy schedule for the all important task of maintaining your health. Somehow you must **make the time.** The consequence of not taking the time now to integrate health practices into your daily life is that you could spend **more** time **not well.** In the long run you are wiser to allot some time now during the week to maintain your health than to pay later with serious time out from a chronic disease that might have been prevented had you maintained your diet, exercise, and meditative practices.

Any change of routine is difficult because we humans are programmed to be creatures of habit. Just remember that once you get your new lifestyle habits in place, they, too, will become difficult to change. Think about how hard it was to remember to brush your teeth as a child. As an adult, brushing your teeth is almost automatic. If you missed a day for some reason, you would probably feel awful!

What competes with your health time?

For most of us the answer would be either work or family plus, of course, television. Because our lives are so complex we seem to be in a constant game of "catch-up". I can tell you that I have things on my "To Do" list that are late by 122 days. Lists do help our feeling that we are in control, but they are not the whole answer. We really must discover where our time goes.

For one day, focus on what you actually do with your time. Look for the places where you can cut a few minutes or longer. For example, I have a policy (not airtight) of keeping my social phone calls down to five minutes or less. I also have learned how to scan newspaper articles instead of reading every word. My television viewing is very limited, but when I do watch television, my sewing kit is nearby, so I can make repairs. I work very hard to keep organized and to plan my activities in advance. But, most importantly I have made my health a top priority.

An activity record

If you really don't know where your time goes may I suggest a simple exercise? For one week keep track of what you are doing, where you are going, and summarize your activity every hour. Use the Activity Record that follows as your blueprint. It is divided into 24 lines, for a 24-hour day with enough room on each line to squeeze in four short words to describe your activities. Each column represents a day of the week. You can bracket the hours together when one activity is spread over a period of hours (for example, sleeping.)

My Activity Record

	MON	TUES	WED	THURS	FRI	SAT	SUN
6:00a.m.							
7:00							
8:00							
9:00							
10:00							
11:00							
12:00p.m.							
1:00							
2:00							
3:00							
4:00							
5:00							
6:00							
7:00							
8:00							
9:00							
10:00							
11:00							
12:00a.m.							

	MON	TUES	WED	THURS	FRI	SAT	SUN
1:00a.m.							
2:00							
3:00							
4:00							
5:00							

Plan ahead

Computers have come to assist us in many ways and one of the best uses of the computer, on a personal level, is that software exists for you to itemize daily tasks and keep a schedule flowing. Decide what hours you have free for scheduling physical play and meditation. Then commit these activities on paper in the appropriate time slot.

If you have no idea where to put exercise, may I suggest finding a time after noon. Recent research suggests that the body may be an afternoon or evening performer. The perceived effort to exercise later in the day is less than the perceived effort to exercise in the morning. Nevertheless your biorhythms could be different. Select the time that feels right for you.

Making lists with or without the assistance of technology helps us to improve our sense of control. And that reduces stress. Finding time in our day can be accomplished, but then you need to find the time to make the plan! Just finding the time to make your new schedule could be challenging! Could you pare down your television viewing to only those programs that are a "must"? Try reading a **printed** television guide first, then do not turn on the television unless there is something you want to watch. If you turn on the television first there is a tendency to switch channels until you find something that is mildly interesting-- and it just consumes time.

Getting birds to fly

Interruptions while you are trying to accomplish a task are one of the most costly time vaporizers. Two interruptions while you are working on a task can make that job take three times as long. Focusing on your work without interruption is optimal. Take note of how you accomplish tasks and what interruptions occur. You may find it necessary to monitor phone calls with an answering machine, and then return calls later. Combining like tasks often saves time. You could also ask friends to call you after a certain time if they are interrupting your business hours.

Difficult as this may be, we all must learn how to say "no" to certain requests. Your time is valuable and by setting your own priorities and goals you will know what activities to eliminate. Whenever I feel overwhelmed I think about the President of the United States and wonder how he (or she someday!) gets the job done. He has lots of help. He even takes vacations. He is highly scheduled. He sets priorities. In a crisis, he drops everything.

Once you can put your schedule on paper it's off your mind. Develop a possible schedule, one you can live with, and reward yourself by checking off tasks as they are accomplished. The biggest anti-depressant is taking action, and one of the best satisfactions is the completion of a task. You will feel good being organized and actually being able to follow your plan.

Once you are able to manage your time, you will also be able to commit to a healthy lifestyle. Losing weight, maintaining weight loss, exercising, and meditating all require some space in time. You could make no better investment.

Time blocks

To organize your day and to be sure that you include time for healthful activities think in terms of blocks of time.

- First, find where your time actually goes. (Complete that Activity Record
- Second, can you delegate some activities to someone else who would do it just as well or better? (your children do their own laundry? Could you trade off food shopping with someone else? Could you service your car at a garage that also washes your car?
- Third, set a block of time aside for no interruptions to get your high priority tasks accomplished.
- Fourth, plan your schedule a week at a time. Allocate some time either at the beginning or end of the week to do this. Make health one of your top priorities on your schedule. Don't sacrifice your health on the altar of work.
- Fifth, follow these basic steps to gain control over your time. Record how you're spending your time now on the activity sheet. Set limits on your activities. For example, if your business meetings take 1 1/2 hours because people are late, be firm about starting on time and keep the meeting to an hour. Work does fill the time available.

Consolidate similar activities. Don't make five trips in the car if you can make one trip to cover all the bases. File your papers at one time or in a consistent manner. Open your mail perhaps at the same time. Put your paper projects together.

Identify your peak work performance hours. Schedule your important tasks then. Identify your low energy times. Schedule easy tasks at those times, or use that time to regenerate with physical play or stress reducing exercises. Time is all we humans really have. Make it count with days where you get out of bed feeling good and love what you see in the mirror.

It's worth your time!

Go to PRACTICE C5 now.

*H*old

● Point 6

Yes, you can eat cake

Are you destined for a life of food group monitoring and palm-portion counting? The answer is yes and no. The purpose of the *MAGIC-HAND* Plan is to teach you how to function like a normally eating person who eats well, but does not gain weight. Since your hand is always with you and you now have been taught to eat "with your eyes" you can go anywhere and use your *MAGIC-HAND.* The system is extremely adaptable to all situations, but you must learn how to use it so that you can live this way and not feel deprived. After you have reached your ideal weight, the challenge facing you is to maintain that weight, that dress or suit size, that wonderful feeling of being light for the rest of your life. While you were losing weight it was necessary to stay strictly with the assigned food groups and portion sizes in order to lose weight. The difference between losing weight and maintaining weight is that when you are losing weight you must choose healthy fiber-rich foods to fit into those palm-portions. For example, your Fruit must be an apple, not a fruitcake! But when you are on maintenance, **after you have reached your ideal weight** and are staying within your ideal weight range, you can opt for more calorie-dense choices-- but still in palm-portions!

It is also possible, when you are maintaining to strictly adhere to the program for (let's say) five days of the week, but not on weekends. You will always be in the program, on the *MAGIC-HAND* Eating Plan, but through trial and error you will discover how much leeway you can take. You will also want to maintain your health so do not stray too far, or take too many liberties from the original plan. Otherwise, you'll be back where you started.

Maintaining-the tricky part

Certainly you can grit your teeth, eat a healthy diet for nine weeks, lose weight, and consider your diet a success. But, the really tricky part, the part that separates the men from the boys, the women from the girls, is **maintaining** that weight loss. In the same breath may I say, that the best part of controlling your weight is not only reaching your goal, but also staying there. Once you have reached your ideal weight, you can start to take some "liberties" with meal planning. Your favorite (calorie-dense) foods can creep back on the menu, but only once in a while and in moderation. You will not have to live without French fried potatoes for the rest of your life! If you see that you are gaining weight again as you add back some calorie-laden foods, and you reach the upper limit of your warning zone, that is the time to get right back on your strict *MAGIC-HAND* Eating Plan.

The most important rule here is never to go two pounds over your ideal weight. (By the same token, don't allow yourself to go two pounds below your ideal weight either.) A two-pound weight gain over your ideal weight is a clear warning that you **MUST** limit or revise your intake again. I'm sorry, but this is the story of our lives. If we didn't have a problem controlling our weight, we could allow free rein-- but we do have this problem. The simple fact is that we-- who want to keep our weight under control-- will be governed by palm-portions for the rest of our lives. As a result we will probably be eating healthier diets and living longer than others. Not a bad sentence!

Stretching palm-portions

Most people enjoy eating an elegant and tasty dessert. I have discovered that everything is in "presentation". Often what separates a high-priced restaurant from the ordinary is the garnish on the plate! Just to give you an idea, here's a suggestion for how you could serve an orange as a sumptuous dessert at home. Take about six orange sections and place them in a dish, arranged like the petals of a flower with ends meeting in the middle. Put a few raisins in the center. Then sprinkle lightly with cinnamon and unsweetened cocoa. Eat with a small fork (and accompanying candlelight). You now have a beautiful dessert- and it can be counted as 1 Fruit chit.

Another way to stretch your palm-portions is to add fruit to whatever you ordinarily might have for dessert. For example, ice cream is a favorite at our house. What I do is to take a half-palm full of fruit, like blueberries, and a half-palm size (about 1 rounded tablespoon) of ice cream and put them both in a dish. I can still count this dessert as one palm-portion, and I feel like I've had a bowl of ice cream, yet I've saved a lot of calories.

If you are someone who likes to indulge in potato chips or tortilla chips, here's a test of your self-discipline. These are high-fat, high calorie foods, so I don't recommend you eat them on a regular basis, but since you're human you just may get the urge. Take a paper towel and place it in front of you. Put your hand in the bag and fill your hand with as many potato or corn chips as you can hold. Place this palm-full on the paper towel and carry it away. (Put the bag back in a cupboard or where you can't see it.) That will be 1 palm-portion of a fatty Carbohydrate.

How can you count alcoholic beverages? If you can visualize the average wine glass half full, that's about 1 chit worth of alcohol. Imagine the liquid fitting in the palm of your cupped hand. It would be between 1/4 to 1/2 cup or about 4-6 ounces. Your judgment and ability to visualize the liquid will enable you to determine the liquid palm-portion. What I do is stretch my palm-portion of alcoholic beverage with water. It's sacrilege to a connoisseur, but I add water to wine and beer-- a not uncommon practice in some European households.

If you enjoy a before-dinner cocktail, how about some vegetable juice on ice with a slice of lemon? It's filling, and doesn't cost one chit. Healthy too.

Do you like hot cocoa? I do. I discovered a way to stretch my palm-portion of milk: I use 1 palm-portion of milk (about 1/3 cup), 1 teaspoon of coffee, 1 tablespoon of Hershey's cocoa (no sugar) and fill with 2/3 cup hot water. Then I add a dash of cinnamon (or vanilla) and I enjoy my cup of hot chocolate.

What about pasta? Do you just love to eat pasta? I do. I am the original spaghetti kid. As a child my mother had difficulty getting me to eat anything else. And it continues to be one of my favorite foods. The way I stretch my pasta is to take a palm-full of pasta (about one ounce- you can weigh it dry), cook it, and then add it to a half bag of cooked frozen string beans or broccoli. (Spaghetti squash works well too.) On top I add a tomato sauce made from tomatoes (no oil) with onions and garlic. I serve with a palm-portion of Parmesan cheese and I've only used 2 chits-- 1 Carbohydrate and 1 Milk. If I add a palm-portion of ground turkey to my sauce I will use another chit for Protein. I have what looks like a plate of pasta and indeed I have fooled myself. After eating, I am very full and satisfied.

With casseroles especially you will find that you have no idea what foods are buried inside. The best thing to do is not to attempt food group dissection. Trade in a palm-portion chit from one of your food groups and serve yourself a palm-potion size of whatever it is, and count it as one chit.

You will soon discover what food group you favor over others. One of my clients told me that her Fruit and Carbohydrate chits always are used first and then she has a hard time getting any Milk products in her diet. If you have plenty of Milk chits remaining, you could use one of those chits for that palm-portion of casserole. You can trade. Just remember that the farther away you get from balancing different food groups, the less healthy is your eating. *MAGIC-HAND* eating makes you very conscious of what you're eating and when you're eating. May I remind you that you should only make trades when you are on maintenance. If you notice any physical change or weight gain, nip it in the bud. You will be amazed at how quickly you can get back to your ideal target. Stay in control. You will discover the joy of maintaining the right weight for your body design and the satisfaction of well-balanced meals.

Juggling chits

We are using the word chit in this book to mean one of your finger palm-portion or thumb servings from a food group. Each day you start with 15 chits (12 palm-portions and 3 thumb-portions). Since this is a forever-eating plan, I recognize that you may want to eat more of one food than another at certain times, deviating from a strict adherence to our guidelines. That's O.K. as long as you trade in your chits from another food group. Let's say that my mother bakes my favorite bread for me and delivers the loaf to my door. Also, let's say it's a trigger food for me. One palm-portion slice won't be enough. I want the whole loaf! Because I have **some** control over my eating, I could trade in my chits from other food groups so that I could have more of the bread. This makes me feel that I will not be depriving myself and that I can have as much as I want as long as I do so in palm-portion sizes and with whatever chits I have remaining. The price I pay is not to have a very well balanced meal plan that day. It's a small price to pay in my opinion for my mother's home baked bread. This is why I am able and you will be able to control your eating using your *MAGIC-HAND* forever. On <u>maintenance</u> you **can** trade in chits from one food group to another.

For people who are on special diets this is a particularly valuable feature of the eating plan. If you are a strict vegetarian you might want to trade in all of your Milk chits for Fruit chits. (You can meet your calcium requirement by eating healthy servings of broccoli and other greens.) Your Protein chits could be used for nuts or grains. You can use the food group chits to complement and balance your proteins, for example, having a palm-portion of rice (Carbohydrate) with a palm-portion of kidney beans (Protein).

Mainly you need to be aware that, in general, whenever you make a trade, while you may be increasing the "livability" of the eating plan, you also may be reducing its health quotient. I call this controlled cheating. If you are a binge eater still struggling to overcome the psychological components of your bingeing, binge in palm-portions not to exceed the allowable limit. This will help you to exercise some control over your compulsion. The next day you might feel sick, but you won't feel as if you "lost it" totally.

Believe me I am not endorsing the behavior, but healing takes time, and regressions are to be expected. If you are trading chits, a good guideline to remember is that one chit (that fits in the palm of your hand) should not exceed 100 calories. If you are not trading chits, don't concern yourself with the calories.

Juggling chits is not advised while you are trying to lose weight since it will slow down the weight-loss process. However, being out of control and overweight is worse.

You may choose on some days to not count your chits. Decide beforehand what occasions these will be and allocate no more than nine days a year. For example, I never count chits on Thanksgiving Day. This does not mean that I go crazy with my eating, but I do eat more. This lets me know that my natural inclinations, left unchecked, are still to gobble! If I ate all that I wanted every day then I wouldn't look the way I want to look. If I want to look slim and feel good, then I have to eat less than I want to eat. It's as simple as that. I am a person who understands your problem. I know what it's like to struggle to keep your weight under control. I am sharing my success with you, and I continue to live what I preach. The truth may be that those of us with a weight problem have a genetic propensity to accumulate fat. Recognizing this fact, we work with what we are given. And we do what we must to counteract our fat accumulation survival trait--to preserve our health in today's world.

Your vote

You may be wondering why I haven't told you not to eat eggs or butter or why I don't seem overly concerned with the specific foods you may choose under each food group category. Certainly I am aware that cholesterol is linked to heart disease, but I am also aware that it is a complicated issue. It depends on the type of cholesterol and even if you get rid of all the cholesterol in your diet, the liver will manufacture its own. The same with salt and blood pressure. Only some people with high blood pressure will get a benefit from reducing the salt in their diet. Whether or not you choose to eat an egg for breakfast I leave as your decision. One egg that fits in the palm of your hand is 1 Protein as far as I'm concerned, and it's an excellent source of vitamins and minerals. What you eat is important, but perhaps **more** important is that you keep your weight under control. Nothing is more devastating to your health than excess body fat.

If you are concerned about your fat intake, I do not discriminate between margarine and butter. With three thumb-joint portions a day I do not think you will be eating too much! If you stay within the food group guidelines you will not be ingesting too much fat from your other foods either. However, once you start making trades, you could eat more than the 30% recommended calories from fat. Remember not all fats are equal. Highly monounsaturated oils such as olive oil, canola and nut oils are believed to contribute to healthy HDL cholesterol levels. Animal fats and other saturated fats may increase unhealthy LDL cholesterol levels. More and more research seems to point in the direction that diet may be a smaller factor than previously thought in lowering serum cholesterol. You be the judge of what foods you want to include in your diet. I am also not going to persuade you to choose foods that are labeled as "low-fat" or as "low cholesterol". If you enjoy the food, if you like the taste, then eat it. It still counts as a 1-

chit portion when you use your *MAGIC-HAND* since we don't count calories. Your low-calorie salad dressing is still a 1 thumb-joint portion chit. I find that I buy both reduced-calorie dressings and other richer dressings, using them both, depending on my mood and desire. I don't worry about gaining weight in either case, since my portions are under control.

While maintaining your ideal weight I would like to persuade you to continue to make healthy food choices. Fresh fruits, fresh vegetables, low-fat or non-animal origin proteins, low-fat milks and cheeses and complex carbohydrates are the best. This demand you should place upon yourself. Educate yourself and please your palate. You are the only person who knows what makes you feel good and healthy.

When I see people substituting some chemical substance for a real egg or using an artificial sweetener I think they are missing the point. These actions do not constitute a healthy lifestyle and are token attempts towards better health. Stay with the real foods, limit your intake, exercise regularly and reduce your stress-- that's the best ticket.

Whether you agree with my philosophy or not, you are free to choose the foods you want to include (even if you insist on chemical eggs). We all make our own choices and your judgment may be different than mine, and your doctor may recommend that you eat specific commercially prepared substitutes. I will not argue. Whatever foods you choose, chemical or real, low-calorie or high-calorie, **IF** you follow the *MAGIC-HAND* Eating Plan, you will lose weight and be able to keep your weight under control. Either way, the program works.

Sweet so-long

There **is** one food that I believe has no value in your diet. That is sugar also known as sucrose, dextrose, and fructose. Sucrose is not metabolized in the body the same way as starch and other complex carbohydrates. Sugars occurring naturally in fruits and vegetables can be handled by the body quite easily whereas refined concentrated sugar can aggravate sensitive pancreatic excretions. The body breaks down white sugar (sucrose) into glucose-- the end product of all the carbohydrate products we eat. When we eat large quantities of sugar, insulin from the islets of Langerhans in the pancreas is secreted into the bloodstream. If the pancreas is over stimulated too much insulin may be secreted. When this happens, the blood sugar level will fall and remain low, possibly causing a craving for more sugar. When people get crotchety or irritated sometimes it's because their blood sugar level is low.

People with hypoglycemia are especially prone to feeling hungry all the time and to becoming easily annoyed at the slightest provocation. Like drug addicts they need a sugar fix. And like drug addicts, the cure is to get unhooked from sugar.

The liver plays a vital function in controlling the normal blood sugar level by removing sugar from and adding sugar to the blood. The activity of the liver is controlled by hormones from the pancreas and adrenal glands. When the adrenal glands are stimulated during periods of strong emotional stress blood sugar levels increase and the result may be hyperglycemia (high blood sugar). When the pancreas can no longer provide insulin, the result is diabetes.

Our body was never designed to handle concentrated forms of sugar. Basically our body has no need for sucrose. When sugar intake exceeds the body's immediate needs, it is quickly converted to fat. Since everyone is genetically different, some people are better able than others to process sweets. If you are overweight, if any blood relative has had diabetes and if you suspect you may have hypothyroidism or a sluggish metabolism, you would be well advised to eliminate or significantly reduce your sugar intake.

Too many foods contain sugar as a "hidden" source of calories. Before foods enter your supermarket basket, read the labels. If sugar is listed as one of the first three ingredients, do not put that item in your basket. The ingredients are listed from high to low, according to the quantity contained. Find another product. You do not need the extra calories from sugar. To keep your intake even to a "moderate" level requires conscientious effort. You find sugar in your food where you least expect it, for example, in ketchup and peanut butter! If you use an artificial creamer in your coffee, probably most of that "milk" is sugar. Very few breakfast cereals contain no sugar-- some have as much as 50 per cent. You sweet tooth is an acquired taste in part. Once you wean yourself from sugar, your taste buds seem to change. What you used to think was just sweet tasting, becomes too sweet--disagreeably sweet. Eliminate refined sugar from your foods. Instead of eating a slice of bread that contains sugar, eat a slice of bread that contains no sugar. (French bread, sour dough and rye bread usually do not have sugar.) Instead of sipping soup that contains sugar, sip soup that contains no sugar. You will not be changing the quantity of food that you eat-- it's still palm size-- but you will be changing the quality. See if you can reduce the amount of sugar in your recipes by half, or use a ripened banana or substitute fruit juice instead. If you were to get rid of every cardboard box, can, frozen package and bottle in your kitchen that contained sugar what would remain? This is a test of how well you have been eating. Replace these items with products that do not contain sugar. If you take just this one step, I guarantee you will lose some weight simply by eliminating the sugar in your diet.

Welcome water

One of the best things you can do for yourself is to drink water. If ever there was an elixir for losing weight, water is it. Water is good for so many things besides a good complexion! Basically water flushes the kidneys. When the kidneys are not fully flushed the liver picks up the extra burden. When the liver is asked to do some of the kidney's work, it cannot optimally do its job of metabolizing fat. Water will also help to rid some of the waste products from the body that were previously stored in your fat cells. As you lose weight, that is- fat, other substances are released into the bloodstream. You want to get rid of these metabolized products as quickly as possible.

While you are losing weight it is important to keep your bowels functioning normally. Water is essential. If your fluids are out of balance constipation results. With adequate water all systems of the body improve. Best of all for most people, with increased consumption of water, their appetite diminishes. Water is filling.

If you do experience hunger while losing weight, here's a little trick that you can do with water to reduce your hunger and appetite: Add a little grape juice (1/4 cup = 1 Fruit chit) to a glass of water and drink it 30 minutes before sitting down to a meal. Whenever you feel hungry, take this little "magic potion" and the physical hunger will subside.

Anyone who knows me can tell you that I am seldom seen without a cup or glass in my hand. During the summer months I have water with a slice of lemon, or one of the flavored mineral waters with ice. During the winter months I have hot water with lemon or an herb tea (non-diuretic). Some teas have a sweet orange spice flavoring that I find substitutes beautifully for dessert. I am always drinking water, hot and cold. I limit the caffeine containing beverages so that I do not lose more water than ingest. Get into the habit of always having a glass or cup of water readily available. And the old adage, to drink at least 8 glasses a day still holds true. Water has no calories. Drink as much as you like. Like Vegetables it is unlimited.

For traveling, keep a plastic container of water with a built in straw or drinking spout. You can take this wherever you go. If your work in an office keep a glass and a pitcher of water on your desk. If you keep your cup, glass or bottle in sight, it will be a natural reminder to drink some water. Drink water before each meal, and after each meal. Instead of snacking while watching television drink a flavored water. It gives you something to do, something to occupy your hands, and something to put in your mouth!

An open hand

The strategy of eating using your hand as a guideline is simple enough. There are indeed some margins for error. You could overestimate how much fits in the palm of your hand. You could make poor food choices. Certainly a brownie as a Carbohydrate is very different than a potato as a Carbohydrate. Milks are different too. There is whole milk, 2% milk and skim milk. I believe that you know that there are more calories in a brownie than in a potato, and that there is more fat in whole milk than in skim milk. But I will not "force" you to drink skim milk, especially if you don't like it. There is no secret about what foods are considered healthy to eat. To lose weight quickly stay with low fat, high fiber, no sugar foods.

However, even if fattier more caloric foods are included, you will **still** lose weight on the *MAGIC-HAND* Eating Plan, but more slowly. This is not a deprivation diet. You can choose the foods you want and make the choice-- to lose weight quickly or more slowly-- by the foods you select in each food group. To maintain your weight loss, you can exercise trading options between food groups, giving yourself even more freedom. Your job is to lose the weight you don't want and to maintain that weight loss.

What makes it possible for you to live with *MAGIC-HAND* eating forever is this built-in flexibility. By monitoring your weight loss, you will discover what liberties you can and cannot take. You will learn how to fine-tune this Plan to your own rhythms of eating. You can trade food groups, and you can spread your meals over the day, eating every hour if you'd like. What stays in place are 12 palm-portions and 3 thumb portions every day, 3 for each food group. You cannot "save" chits from one day to use for another. Nor are you required to use all your chits if you don't feel like eating. Every day starts with 12 palm-portions and 3 thumb-joint portions.

Within the rules of this Eating Plan, you have full control over what you eat, when you eat and how often you eat. Give the illusion of being one of the skinny people who eats what he or she wants--the *illusion* of not controlling, of not being on a diet, when in fact you are. Is this Plan too permissive for you or will it enable you to live a life of pleasure-- **in control** of maintaining your ideal weight? I have dared to remove the handcuffs. I trust that you know what's good for you.

Variety is the spice of life!

Go to PRACTICE H6 now.

*A*dapt

● Point 7

This is a road show

One of the benefits of having an eating plan tied to your hand is that it is something that travels with you wherever you go. Most lose-weight programs do not permit the degree of freedom and flexibility offered by the *MAGIC-HAND* Eating Plan. This program is lifelong therefore it **must** be livable and it must be able to accommodate all the influences, pitfalls, and assaults coming from outside your home. In society at large, the dieter is constantly challenged. That means no matter where you are-- in a plane, at your mother's house or at a weenie roast-- you can still eat and not gain weight if you follow the principles of *MAGIC-HAND* eating.

One of our basic tenets is that you should not feel deprived while living with your *MAGIC-HAND*. In this point we will discuss how you can have your cake, eat it, and not gain weight. Eating outside your home does not mean that you have no control over your situation. One by one we'll tackle the most common social situations where overeating is sanctioned and even encouraged. You will have to learn how to cope in these situations where so many of the "right" foods are not available and it is time to eat.

Where most of us have difficulty controlling our intake is over the winter holidays, traveling, and eating at restaurants. Are you ready to learn the tricks of the slim people? Let's begin our journey out there in the world of eating booby traps.

Fast-food dilemma

Especially if you travel on the road, or have children, fast-food restaurants are hard to ignore. They are convenient, efficient, and inexpensive. More and more fast-food restaurants are starting to offer healthier options and may include a salad bar or broiled chicken. You can balance your meal using palm-portions. For example, an order of milk, a small burger and a side salad with dressing will probably cost you four palm-portions and a thumb of oil, but you'll be eating from all the food groups, and thereby still be on the Plan. Hopefully you will feel full and satisfied.

Calorie-laden fast foods are to be consumed judiciously, and infrequently, and must be made accountable for the amount of fat, protein, and carbohydrate they contribute to your well-balanced diet. If you cannot balance your meal at a fast-food restaurant and you eat more than a palm-portion, you can compensate at the next meal by eating less than a palm-portion in that food group (and fill your plate with a large serving of greens).

Traveling on wheels

Maintaining your weight is a heroic challenge for the constant traveler. You are at the mercy of roadside restaurants, train dining or snack cars, and in-flight menus.

When you are on the road, you lack control over your general diet-- therein lies the problem. But, you can put the odds in your favor. Try to keep your meals regular by not skipping any meals. Some foods you can keep supplied in your own car. You'll save money if you keep some tangerines in your car and have one as your breakfast fruit instead of ordering a glass of fruit juice. They keep well and are tasty and filling. Or, you could keep a six-pack of fruit juice. If you will be traveling for two or more hours in the car, you would be well advised to keep what I call a "snack pack". A quick snack can prevent you from having to stop at a fast-food place because you are hungry. Sometimes a half-hour on the road means the difference between stopping at a greasy-spoon type of place or stopping at a place that might serve a healthier menu.

Your portable snack pack could include canned vegetable or fruit juice, sunflower seeds or nuts, peanut butter on crackers, small boxes of raisins, breadsticks or crackers, tea or coffee and a small bottle of mineral water. All these foods will "keep" for a while and do not require refrigeration. I maintain a pack like this in my car for emergencies, and I regularly replace the older food items. It has saved me many times from having to purchase foods in desperation when I felt hungry. I also know that what I'm eating is healthier than the average road fare. That's a real plus.

In the air

Many airlines give you a choice of several menus and often there is a "lighter" menu. Using your finger-palm, thumb-joint method you can keep your portions under control no matter what you select. En route, generally you are offered soft drinks, alcoholic beverages, mineral water or club soda, milk, tea, coffee, and fruit or vegetable juices. The smart choices are non-dehydrating beverages like mineral water and fruit and vegetable juices or milk. If you order mineral water or a vegetable juice you don't have to give up any chits. And, of course, you could have as much tea or coffee as you'd like, but they tend to be dehydrating. Select your foods carefully and count your beverage consumption as part of your meal. Remember that you are not required to eat everything put in front of you.

On solid turf

The problem with eating at restaurants is that in general they serve too much food! All the food groups are likely to be represented, offering you the possibility for a balanced meal. To get variety into my diet, I order at restaurants those foods I don't usually prepare at home (or are difficult to prepare tastefully). Rather than to order a full meal, depending on your circumstances, soup and salad and a slice of French bread might be enough. Do not feel compelled to order the complete dinner. If others are ordering the dinner special, you can ask for your salad first and also ask for the soup to be served at the time of the entrees. Ordering a la carte is a way for you to plan your own meal. Just say to the waitperson, " I'll have my soup as the entree." If your companions want to know why you're not having a full dinner, don't say you're watching your weight. Simply say, "Soup and salad are just my favorite thing." Or, "I feel like having a light supper, so I'm going to have the soup and salad."

But, you might want to order from the regular dinner menu. You are probably aware that most restaurants still consider meat to be the center of attention, so your protein portion will be larger in most instances than the palm of your hand. Rather than to over-indulge and put on weight that you don't want, follow these simple guidelines:

- immediately, when your entree arrives, take your knife and fork and cut the meat portion in half (assuming it is twice the size of a palm-portion). Make believe that one half of it doesn't exist and put it to the side of your plate. You **can** eat the other half.

- Eat all your vegetables and the salad- they are "unlimited", but be careful about how much dressing you use. One tablespoon of salad dressing would be one thumb-joint of salad oil. A pat of butter on your slice of bread would also be a one thumb-joint chit. So, keep counting. If you planned properly during the day, you should have enough chits left (because you saved some) to be able to eat this dinner. At the end of the meal, when the waitperson returns, ask for the doggie bag and the meat/protein portion that you didn't eat may find itself in tomorrow's lunch or dinner. (This technique will also save you money!)
- Peruse the dessert menu and decide if anything on that menu is appealing enough to use yet another palm-portion chit. Some desserts are larger than a palm-portion, and even if they fit within the palm of your hand, desserts tend to be rich (over 100 calories) so if you really want something on the menu ask if someone else at the table would be willing to split a dessert with you because you are just too "full" to have a whole one. Most restaurants these days are very accommodating and will even bring you an extra fork and plate. Do not feel forced to order dessert because everyone else does. You can say, "That cheesecake sounds so good, but I'm so full, I think I'll just have coffee." Say it with a smile. Tell yourself that you are full and can't eat any more. If you still have a palm-portion chit left after your dinner, you could have dessert, but it is not a requirement. If you feel full, and you will not feel deprived by not having dessert, I'd say you're better off without it. Because of the hidden sugars and fats, even if you have not over-indulged at your favorite restaurant, you probably have ingested more calories than you would ordinarily at home.

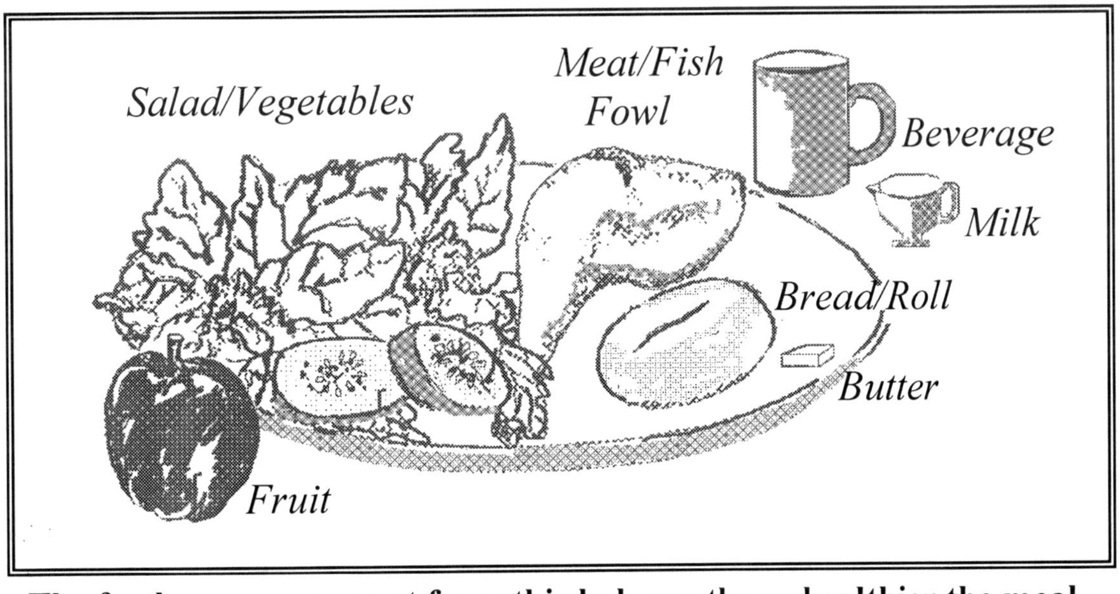

The farther away you get from this balance the unhealthier the meal.

Keep in mind the example of an ideal meal: Two to four ounces of animal or vegetable protein-- the protein that fits in the palm of your hand; one slice of bread or a roll, one pat of butter, and any amount of raw or fresh or slightly cooked vegetables and a piece of fruit and perhaps a small glass of milk. That's a lot of food and you do not need to eat everything at one sitting. It's best to eat as you feel hungry.

Take your hand with you and plan ahead for eating at restaurants by cutting back some of your chits from other meals. Portion control is the essence of successful restaurant eating. Just because you are at a restaurant doesn't mean that you can throw caution to the wind. Consider it another meal, the main reason for being there is probably to be with other people, not to eat. Eating-out is a challenge that you can overcome with your *MAGIC-HAND*. Enjoy the outing, enjoy the company, enjoy the surroundings, and enjoy being in control as you place your order. Think of how happy you will be when you've not gained weight.

At a restaurant tonight's dinner is also tomorrow's lunch. Start by cutting your main entree in half. Don't be afraid to "doggie bag"-- even the potatoes and bread.

HANDling the holidays

They come but once a year, at the end of the year, starting at Thanksgiving and ending on New Year's Day at which time we resolve to lose all the weight we gained. During the other months of the year, January through October there are also feast days available to us, but nothing as consistent and overbearing as during November and December. The word holiday in itself predicts behavior. It's a day of freedom from "whatever". Often that translates into a day of freedom to do as I please: laugh hard, play hard, and well-- eat, eat, eat-- as much as I want. And the food is available almost everywhere you go. Stores have samples, offices have special treats, almost every organization and business has a party, and relatives send fruit cakes and cookies. It's no wonder that the average person gains from 4 to 7 pounds over the holiday months.

You and I who love to eat are forced into this situation whether we like it or not. So we must do battle to protect our svelte figures. We are armed with our hand! Does this mean we can never eat a meal without counting palm-portions? No, it does not.

Most often during the holidays we are invited to cocktail parties and big dinners or big buffets. Everyone is expected to eat and enjoy. To keep on the *MAGIC-HAND* Eating Plan it is necessary to plan your day's eating when you know that you will go out later to a party. Generally what I do is "save chits". I eat a light breakfast, I eat a light lunch and then with my extra chits (palm-portions) I can eat more than I ordinarily would at a party-- but I am still counting palm-portions. I bring my hand with me and I know for that evening I can have 8 palm-portions because I saved some chits from meals earlier in the day. Usually I try to predict or spy the dessert and determine if I need to save a chit for that. I only eat desserts that I like! I do not attempt to try to balance my food groups at a party, but I will eat as many vegetables as I can because I know they are unlimited and they are filling. If you know that a big dinner will be served, don't overindulge on hors d'oeuvres. Eat the carrot sticks, zucchini slices and if you lace them in a dip, count a tablespoon of dip as 1 Oil/Fat chit.

In general, try to avoid the hot fried hors d'oeuvres. Nibble on raw vegetables if possible. And before you sit down to eat keep in mind your finger-palm foods and how you will carefully select the foods to enjoy. It's never a good idea to arrive at the dinner table feeling "starved". Spread your eating throughout the day or eat 1 Fruit or snack on vegetables about 30 minutes ahead of the feast to curb your appetite.

Before I go to a party or dinner I will know how many chits I have left for the day so I might leave the house with 2 thumbs of Oils/fat and 6 palm-portions of Milk/ Fruit/Carbohydrate/Protein remaining. I can remember how many chits I have left and as I eat I say to myself "There goes one thumb, I have one thumb left. There goes 2 palm-portions, I still have 4 left." With planning and practice you will become quite skilled at parceling out your portions. Since you probably will have no idea what is in the casserole you're eating or the doctored sweet potatoes or maybe even what the main entree is, do not bother to try to balance the meal. Just eat what you want, but count the finger-palms and thumbs! For example, a palm-portion of a casserole dish would be whatever might fit in the cupped palm of your hand. If you are not serving yourself and the hostess places more on your plate than a palm-portion, leave it on the plate or eat it all, but count an extra chit. Get it? Count your half glass of wine as a chit.

At the cocktail party count whatever you drink as a chit if it is about a half-cup liquid. Better, however, is to forego the alcohol, and ask for a Virgin Mary (tomato juice with lemon) or a V-8. This way you can save a chit (palm-portion) for dinner or an appetizer. You must also learn how to say, "No, thank you." Never ever say that you are on a diet. Once you say that EVERYONE will want you to eat. From my own observations, people can accept "I am full." "I am saving myself for dessert." "I'm just not a pumpkin pie fan. Thank you." "I'd love to, but I'm allergic to strawberries." "Oh, I'm stuffed." "I just can't eat any more." But, say "I'm on a diet." and your host or hostess will not leave until you have a piece! They say things like, "Oh, a little bit won't hurt. It's my favorite chocolate recipe." Then where are you? If you still say no, it's almost like insulting your host or hostess.

Learn the phrases of the skinny people. You will discover that many of them are "full" or "will have some later" or "already had some and it was great"

Here are some more skinny phrases. During cocktails when appetizers are offered, say "Thank you, but I'm saving myself for dinner." "Thank you, but we're going out for dinner later." Then, at dinner, you can politely decline second helpings by saying, "Thank you, but I'm saving myself for dessert." Then, when the dessert arrives, you can say either "Oh, just a little piece, I'm stuffed." or "I'd like some, but I'm just too full."

Sometimes food is just placed in front of you. In these situations, you must learn to leave the food on your plate. Count your palm-portions, decide how you want to use them and leave the rest! Just say, "I'm so full, I can't finish it all." Whatever you do, don't try to explain how you're limiting your foods now because you're trying to lose weight or get healthy-- it's downright boring. Finish your meal with coffee or tea if served, and you can have seconds and thirds of that!

Plan for "after-dinner" parties in the same way. Modify your intake at dinner. Eat "just a little bit" (whatever chits you have saved) and make it last. Keep the food on your plate as long as you can while you talk, taking small bites. Again, we are not concerning ourselves with balancing food groups, just with keeping the number of portions within your daily allotment. In general, it's a good idea to eat slowly at every meal.

The coffee klatch

Part of "tradition" seems to be donuts for everyone at the office, and at home, to supply coffee cake with the coffee. Again, you must learn to say no to these food complements or you must learn how to trade one palm-portion from one of your healthy food groups.

If you work in an office bring in a bag carrots, put them in a vase of water, and eat one whenever you're hungry. Let them all laugh, and let them eat the cake. You'll be looking beautiful while they make dental appointments. Soon they may follow your lead.

Partying

How can you have cocktails without hors d'oerves? Or, go to a cocktail party and not have a cocktail? I think by now you may know the answer to these two questions. For cocktail parties, stay with the vegetable appetizers-- slices of zucchini, carrots, mushrooms and celery-- if available. You really do not want to spoil your appetite for dinner! If there is someone tending bar there is often no problem. If your host is the bartender and asks for an explanation you can say, as I do, "I tend to fall asleep with alcohol." "Or, alcohol makes me sleepy." No one wants a sleepy guest at a party!

Always go to a party with at least five-- five finger-palm/thumb portions. If I bring my hand with me and I know I can have five finger-palm/thumbs, it's easy to count. As I serve myself I can do so in tablespoons. I know that for me about 2 tablespoons equals 1 palm-portion. I can also visualize foods on my plate in tablespoons if I don't want to position my palm over the food. I love going to parties with my *MAGIC-HAND* because it's my secret weapon. People usually tell me how wonderful I look and they see that I'm eating the same food they are. They wonder how I keep so slim. It's with my sleight of hand! (You and I know.)

Guesting

Where you really lack control is in someone else's home! What can you do when you are served glazed donuts for breakfast? Your best friends may eat this way and think it's just fine. You could marvel at the donuts and say how wonderful they are but you're a light morning eater and could you have toast and milk instead. (Most households have bread and milk on hand.) Your host or hostess is usually trying to please **you**, so feel free to ask for what you'd like. Survey the kitchen to see if there is any fruit in sight. You can also stack the odds in your favor by bringing a "house present"-- perhaps a basket of fruit and cheese. You can suggest placing it in the kitchen and if they don't open it, say, "Would you mind if I opened the basket and we can see how good these apples are?" Again, don't mention that you're watching your weight. No one needs to know. This is your challenge: to eat well, to maintain your weight, and to use your *MAGIC-HAND* under all circumstances and conditions. Of course, if your hostess serves you a homemade cake, made in your honor, you may be "obliged" to be "polite". If you really like the cake, take one piece and eat as much as would fit in the palm of your hand, leave the rest on your plate claiming that your eyes were bigger than your stomach. (Perhaps it could even be saved for you in the refrigerator either to take home or for later.) Count the palm-sized serving as 1 Carbohydrate.

If you plan to be at another's home for an extended period of time, you might ask your host or hostess, "Would it be easier for you to shop if I told you what I generally like to eat?" Or, you could offer to go shopping with them (because you love to explore new supermarkets). Whenever my husband and I visit our relatives we always ask if we can tag along on a food-shopping trip. We generally enjoy seeing new places and it also gives us an opportunity to share in some of the expenses. We have fun, and in my opinion, it's one of the best ways to get a sense of the community and see the people who live there.

As a guest, you are privileged to make some special requests, keeping in mind and considering the lifestyle of your hosts. But, even your best intentions can be foiled. I remember asking for peanut butter, thinking I couldn't go too far wrong with that request. I was wrong. The hostess returned with a sugared jellied peanut butter swirl. The **second** ingredient in the peanut butter was sugar! It was awful. I've lost my sweet tooth, but I did try to eat some of it. As a result I learned my lesson and whenever I stay for an extended period of time in someone else's home, I try to include myself in their food shopping activities or volunteer to do the shopping. Truly, there is no place like your own home.

In a nutshell

Plan for parties and special events by modifying your intake (saving chits) at other meals during the day. You cannot save up chits from a previous day or not eat as much the next day. Every day must stand on its own two feet and be governed by your hand! The rule is: twelve finger-palm food portions and three thumb-joints a day, and unlimited vegetables.

Everyone has their own way of modifying their intake. Some people skip breakfast, which I don't recommend if it makes you "too hungry". For after-dinner parties I usually forego one milk and my starch and fat at dinnertime anticipating the foods that are likely to tempt me at a party. For dinner I'll have my protein portion and an almost full plate of vegetables which I find very satisfying and filling. (I may drink some milk just before I leave for the party if it will take the edge off of any "hunger".). Then I can eat just "a little bit" for appearances sake. I will eat the starch that fits in the palm of my hand. This could mean some crackers or puff pastry. You **can** make trades and once you become practiced in the system, your eating habits can be easily governed.

Inevitably you will encounter people who encourage you to eat even when they know that you are in the process of losing weight. Prepare yourself for dealing with these saboteurs. These people are engaging in a thinly veiled power struggle to break down your resolve. Recognize it for what it is and resolve to win. If this person is your husband, wife or someone else close to you it may suggest that there are other power issues that need to be addressed as well. You need to put the control and power on your side when it comes to eating. Let them "win" somewhere else if it's that important, but not on **your** plate!

Fast-food restaurants, dinner dates, traveling, partying, and coffee klatches won't throw you off your diet any more. Beware of strange places and use your head as well as your hand. Because this Plan is adaptable, excesses of food, family, and accompanying feelings at social events outside your home can be safely negotiated. It takes practice.

Minefields ahead!

Go to PRACTICE A7 now.

Nurture

● Point 8

The magic power of meditation

Stress, physical or psychological, can wear you down. Simply defined stress is any condition that impinges upon the organism, requiring an adjustive reaction. Selye defines stress as "the non-specific response of the body to any demand placed upon it ". It is any change--positive or negative-- that requires adjustment or adaptation.

Nurturing is the antidote to stress. It is any supportive environment that contributes to survival-- ones ability to adjust and adapt. Quiet time or meditation provides the stage for decompression, for a natural restoration of calm. Physical exercise is also an antidote to stress. At the right level, exercise produces a degree of protection against stress. Neuromuscular tension can be relieved through physical activity. On the other hand, physical over-exertion, just like emotional stress, can exhaust the body, making one again susceptible to illness. The key is to exercise intelligently--moderately-- so that the body remains in the stage of resistance, built up to cope with stress and ward off disease.

The symptoms of too much stress (over-exertion and tension) cause the distress of depression, fatigue, backache, loss of sleep, losing or gaining weight, irritability, headaches and a variety of immune system-related illnesses. Stress from physical exertion due to too much exercise can result, in some cases, in total physical collapse.

The most common stress, however, is the emotional tension that at day's end leaves us tired. If you feel drained much of the time, get colds whenever they are going around, and lack the motivation to stay with a health program, you may need an antidote to either physical or emotional stress.

Challenge

Environmental challenges to our bodies and psyches can be beneficial or harmful. Some physical and mental stress is necessary to keep us well. Too little stress, called "underload" creates boredom and frustration resulting in the same ailments as "overload". People enjoy challenges and generally are motivated to achieve, accomplish, and to succeed. Too much striving, however, can throw us off balance and our bodies scream "Halt!" If we pay no heed we're likely to get sick. That's one way our body enforces "Stop."

The endocrine system of ductless glands (which includes the pituitary, adrenals, thyroid, parathyroid, sex glands, and the pancreas) interacts with the nervous system to bring about homeostatic responses of the body. Stressful situations tax both the nervous and endocrine systems-- essentially the two systems that coordinate the physiological functions of the human organism. And if the stressor persists, the organism may be forced beyond the limits of its ability to adapt. At any rate, there is no doubt that high levels of emotional tension increase one's susceptibility to illness.

Stress if not managed can lead to ulcers, heart attacks, and other diseases. Stress, if managed, can keep you alive and vigorous, enjoying the pleasures and challenges of life. So, how can we cope with the stressors in our lives?

Concerns about our love-life, work situation and money probably account for most, if not all, the emotional stress in our everyday living. Many live in fear of failing in all three. Others know how to find peace. At home do you find love? At work do you find satisfaction? And in your checking account do you find enough money to pay your bills? Examine these three arenas and observe when you feel frustrated, angry or depressed.

Heartstrings

It's true. Happy lovers do live longer. Unresolved, uncertain and difficult love relationships can harm your health. In a study of stress-related illnesses, various life change events were analyzed for their impact on health. The three events at the top of the list--showing the greatest impact on health--were death of a spouse, divorce, and marital separation. Change, whether it is good or bad for you, is stressful to the biological organism and stress can make you more susceptible to the onslaught of disease. Loss of a loved one is especially traumatic. We fear disappointment in love and are reluctant to take the risk of entering into love relationships-- we have the "fear of losing". Though there is no greater stress than the disruption of an established relationship, there is also no greater reward (or calm) than the continuation of a mutually satisfying relationship. Love is a double-edged sword. With love, you can combat stress and conquer fear.

Good friends, like caring lovers, are invaluable resources in life. Married people and people with good friends, sharing a sense of community, live longer than those who are uncoupled or friendless. For the many centenarians living in the Republic of Georgia, a person's wealth is determined by the number of human relationships she or he can establish and maintain. With love and with friendship you can light up your life.

The physical side of love also keeps us healthy. From touching and hugging to sexual intercourse, there are real body benefits: deeper breathing, increased stimulation and circulation. Even a tender embrace can have an astonishing therapeutic effect. Touching is so important to our well-being that infants deprived of tactile stimulation, although well nourished, will become sickly and die. Hugging is an antidote for stress. And the stimulation associated with sexual excitement and intercourse appears to be a tonic for the entire body. With an increase in sexual tension, the heartbeat quickens, blood pressure rises, muscle tension increases, hyperventilation occurs and the blood supply is increased to all parts of the body. Then orgasm brings release and the body returns to a calmer, more relaxed state. At any age, sex can work wonders. Allow your mind and body to relax in the luxury of love.

Breathe in love and exhale stress.

Working well

Stressful jobs tend to be those with long working hours that are either fast paced or filled with repetitive boring tasks. Many service-oriented jobs are high-stress jobs. Secretaries and nurses, because much is demanded of them and they have very little control over their environment, lead the list of individuals in stressful jobs. If you can manage your job stress, it will keep you alive and vigorous. You will have turned a burden into a benefit and your job will be a pleasure and a challenge, a source of healthful stimulation. Some mothers with small children feel exhilarated, while others are ready to "throw in the towel". The former manage the stress of infant care while the latter crumble beneath it.

We must learn to listen to our inner stirrings. A job that nurtures you is fulfilling and rewarding. You have more energy at the end of the day than you had at the beginning. A job that depletes you is one that takes away your energy and leaves you empty. (And food may be filling that spot.)

One of my first jobs after I finished graduate school was a middle management position for a county health service. I was constantly frustrated because I felt the tremendous responsibility of the job but did not have the authority to implement solutions to problems. It was at this time in my life that I had to take the most sick leave from work. I also experienced vision problems, developed dental problems, and gained weight rapidly. (Subconsciously, my added weight gave me the "authority" I needed!)

A frustrating job fraught with tension will wreak havoc with your well-being. You may find it necessary to change jobs or to restructure your present job to maintain your health and sanity. I know such things are easier said than done, but your future health, your well-being, your happiness and your longevity depend upon your actions today.

Tell your boss when a demand is unreasonable. Set realistic deadlines for yourself. Structure your job so you can get the satisfaction that success brings. Also take time during the workday to relax. In between phone calls, roll your head and neck in a circle almost touching your shoulders. And spend a few moments enjoying the release of tension.

During your lunch break (or coffee break or in the rest room) rest your eyes. Sit quietly, close your eyes, and simply cover them with the palms of your hands. Your hands are stress-reducing tools too! This exercise, called "palming", should be done in a comfortable position--with your elbows supported and with your neck in line with your backbone. Loosely cup your palms over your eyes and enjoy this sweet warm rest. In about ten minutes, having stimulated the circulation by relaxing your eyes, you will be ready to return your eyes to work.

Another excellent antidote to stress is oxygen. When you feel overwhelmed by the stress and tension of your work and you need quick relief, reach for oxygen. Stop whatever you are doing, collect yourself, and take three long, slow, deep breaths. And when you are about to face a potentially stressful situation, these long, deep breaths can prevent tension build up. The next time your boss calls you into his office (or your child has dumped a sack of flour on the kitchen floor) pause before you act; breathe deeply and allow the oxygen to bring you calm. It takes only a few seconds and it works.

To the bank

When you don't have money to take to the bank, money becomes an overriding concern. Our feelings of security and control can be undermined by a lack of money. Don't allow life to take you. Stay in control; be the master. If you are pressured by money problems you are either spending more than you have or want more than you can afford. Live within your means and if necessary learn to do without. Get rid of your charge cards, place a restriction on any new purchases, sell any extraneous possessions you can bear to part with, and one by one pay the outstanding bills until you can relax once again.

Take charge of financial matters by writing down and itemizing your outstanding debts, plans for payment, and expected future income. This simple act will reduce your financial problems to a sheet of paper. They may not go away immediately, but the facts and figures will be there for you to analyze. By exteriorizing, you de-emotionalize them-- what seemed overwhelming in your imagination becomes something you can analyze and hope to control. The very process of writing down a problem and listing potential solutions can reduce stress. This process is especially helpful if you find yourself unable to sleep at night. The proper place for a problem is on a sheet of paper. You can quite literally put it away before you go to bed and get it out again for further consideration at an appropriate time later.

It is virtually impossible to eliminate all stress from your life, but you can learn to manage stress. Feeling **in control** is key. Of course, we are all different. What is stressful for one person, may be a healthy challenge for another.

Clearing the mind

The prolonged stresses associated with daily living can sap us of our energy. Here are some ways to keep an even keel and take the wind out of the sails of stress. We can (1) change our perspective on life, (2) structure our days to gain control, (3) build up our resistance to fatigue by maintaining good health, and (4) nourish our psyches through meditation.

● (1) Develop a perspective on life that allows you to focus on life's rewards and take its pains in stride. Learn to choose which stresses you will react to and to differentiate between large and small ones. A late appointment is a small stress while the loss of a family friend or favorite pet is significant. These situations do not deserve the same emotional intensity-- don't give it to them.

You can overcome the small stresses by acknowledging that they are exactly that-- small stresses. What's the point of getting angry if your date is a half hour late for lunch? Anger won't shorten the wait. It will only raise your blood pressure, making you the victim. If you're left waiting for a half hour, you can choose to get upset or to pass it off lightly. And don't worry about the "wasted time"-- you can do some pelvic tilt exercises while you're waiting! So, sigh a deep sigh, breathe in that oxygen and put a smile on your face. Then decide when late is "too late" and relieve yourself of the obligation of waiting any longer. Laugh at your predicament, eat your lunch, and take advantage of this opportunity to be alone with your thoughts. Maintain a sense of humor and don't give events more importance than they deserve. Should your lunch date appear when you're half way through your meal, feel free to leave when you're finished. Take care of yourself. Your time is valuable. And be aware that others may not be considerate-- a reflection on them. If so, you don't need these people in your life!

Another small stress that often becomes major is fighting traffic. My teeth used to clench, my heart pound, and my blood pressure rise every time I was caught in a traffic jam. Then one day I realized that instead of being annoyed, I could use the delay to collect my thoughts or tune in a favorite station on the radio or play a cassette. I realized I had control over my own reactions. Now, when I'm in that stop and go traffic, I breathe deeply, look around me, and smile. I know it's one of those small stresses that doesn't deserve a lot of my energy, so I might as well sit back, relax and enjoy the extra travel time. Simply some things are out of your control. Recognize when they are. Allow extra time if you can when traveling on the road. It usually pays.

Save your angst for the major stresses that come to us simply in the course of living and loving. The loss of a loved one is difficult for most of us to handle. In this situation acknowledge that you are facing a highly stressful, major life change. Allow yourself the full range of emotion-- go ahead and cry, feel sad, experience your grief. Putting up "a good front" will only add to the tension. During this healing time, you may find spiritual communication, the love of others and quiet times by yourself most beneficial. Keep your life at status quo-- "on hold"-- until you recover from the trauma. Resist the temptation to follow the advice of well-meaning friends who suggest yet other major life changes as a cure. Pull in your horns and come out when you're ready.

● (2) Many small stresses can be structured away. We gain control over our lives by organizing our time, planning a schedule and writing things down-- be it in a calendar book, a list of "things to do" or a five-year business plan. Assign priorities to your activities and don't overcrowd the agenda. Structure your days and see to it that every day includes some "free time". If you get fun out of reading poetry (or drawing cartoons, or reading mail order catalogues, or arranging flowers), do that during your free time. Do something for joy. Every day should have some fun time along with those stressful uncontrollable moments we all face. Structure your days, weeks and months to give yourself those fun times-- after all you are the one in charge of your own time.

● (3) Of course, the best defense against being worn down by stress is a good offense. Good health and physical fitness give you staying power to cope with life's challenges. Prolonged stress can lead to exhaustion, resulting in sickness, but a healthy body has reserves.

When you feel your body tensing, shake it out. Wiggle your arms, legs and head. Any physical activity will be helpful. And lack of physical activity can be detrimental. The next time you are tense, go for a walk and see how much better you feel.

Discover what soothes you. Our rewards are those activities which nourish the self. We can relieve stress by physically indulging ourselves (I don't mean eating!): bathing in a hot tub, sitting by the fire, relaxing in the sun or in a sauna, napping while wrapped in warm towels, getting massaged, or listening to music-- a rhythmic soothing melody.

● (4) The healing silence of meditation can restore your health and vitality. The physiological benefits of meditation have been well documented.

...the conscientious practice of meditation increases autonomic ability, aids in habituation to repeated stresses, and produces a state of relaxation deeper in some respects than that induced during sleep. In addition, the characteristic physiological pattern of a person during meditation is virtually opposite to that of a neurophysiological stress pattern. These effects of meditation can carry over and extend into the post meditation stage of daily activity ...K.R. Pelletier.

Meditation is a simple way to relax, a way to find quiet time-- there's nothing mysterious about it. In meditation, your goal is to reach an alpha state brain rhythm and to clear your mind of all thought. The purpose is to achieve a peaceful inner calm and balance in your life. Techniques of meditation are offered here for your experimentation.

Find the one that appeals to you the most or develop your own.

Yogis meditate by devoting their attention solely to their breathing. In a lotus position, legs crossed and back erect with palms open, they focus on the two tones of breathing-- in and out-- referred to as "sa" and "hum". Some meditate using a mantra, which is a word or sound repeated over and over again. Popular word sounds are those with "m" sounds, like "om" believed by some to be a healing vibration. Reciting this mantra sweeps away other thought. The purpose of focusing attention on either breathing or a mantra is to achieve inward centering. Oddly enough, watching television can also produce an alpha state and bring relaxation, that is, if you don't involve yourself with the program but simply allow the sounds and motions to occupy your mind, excluding other thought.

The meditation I recommend is particularly well suited to practicing before you go to sleep. It allows you to dissolve depression, aggravation and tension by sending your troubles away.

Triple phase power meditation

Get yourself into a comfortable position with your back straight either sitting in a chair or lying on the floor with knees bent, feet on the floor. Close your eyes and breathe slowly and deeply. You are now ready to experience the three phases in this meditative process: disposing of the past, becoming aware of the present and relaxing the muscles of your body.

Phase 1.

The purpose of the first phase is to bring yourself to the present by disposing of the past. While you are relaxed with eyes closed and hands clasped across your midsection focus on the events of the day. Watch yourself arise in the morning, eat breakfast, get dressed, etc.-- follow your actions throughout the day. View the events of the day as if you are watching a silent movie. Do not dwell on problematic parts of the day or delve into meanings. Think only in terms of events. For example, if you have an argument don't relive the emotional warfare. Say to yourself "And then I saw Sally and we had an argument and then I left the supermarket with the groceries for supper tonight", etc. Observe yourself with emotional detachment. If you find an event particularly disturbing, label it as a "bad scene" or "a disruptive mess". Go on and bring yourself right up to your present place by reciting the most recent events. For example: "I hung up my clothes, put on my nightgown, brushed my teeth and now I am here lying in bed." Take the day, wrap it in a package, tie it with a knot or bow and throw it away. The day is over and you are here now. Tomorrow will be a new day and you must clear the day.

Phase 2.

Place your arms alongside your body, hands relaxed, palms up. This time is for "nothing". The day is gone. What remains is the now: peace and calm. With your palms facing the sky, it can also be an inspirational or spiritual time. It is a time to receive, to be here. Lie quietly, with no thoughts, until you feel "full". Tune in to the rhythm of your breathing. Enjoy the pleasure of being.

Phase 3.

Bring your hands back to a clasped position over your stomach. . Go over your entire body from head to toe and see if you can't identify some tense places. Then, RELAX. Go through your body again from toes to head. Any muscle that you find that feels tense, RELAX. Breathe. Visualize your body as relaxed and at your ideal weight. Affirm to yourself: "I am ...... pounds (insert the number). Go through your body and see your ideally well-defined figure.

This meditation is one I developed to combine clearing the mind, relaxing the body, and using affirmations. It is a "hybrid" combining several different approaches. Feel free to add or alter the components as you wish. It must serve you. Practice your meditation at any time of the day. If you are a person who has difficulty getting to sleep, meditation is particularly good to practice before going to bed.

The Triple-Phase-Power meditation should be practiced every day for at least 15 to 20 minutes. It will help you to more easily adapt to the many lifestyle changes we are introducing-- changes in eating habits and changes in exercise.

We know that any change in your life pattern-- whether it brings pain or pleasure, benefit or harm-- is likely to bring stress as well. And we also know that habits are nature's way of incorporating efficient behaviors into that pattern. When you do something automatically, having made it a habit, you conserve energy, save time and avoid stress.

Transforming new behaviors into habits is a gradual process, and it usually works best if only one or two new behaviors are introduced at a time. It's estimated to take a consistent 21 days of practicing the new behavior to form a habit. Organize and simplify your life, making room for your psyche to absorb changes-- gradually with a minimum of stress.

Again, try to simplify your life and incorporate changes one at a time. For example, when you are about to have visitors from out-of-town, don't decide to hire an interior decorator to go over a new plan for the living room. The impact of your visitors on you lifestyle is enough stress for the week. Find the calm periods in your life to introduce change.

The peace of meditation will give you the support you need to accomplish the changes in lifestyle that you desire, comfortably, easily.

Look at the glass as half full. And take a big drink.

Give yourself a break!

Go to PRACTICE N8 now.

Daily

● Point 9

The long view

You say you want to lose weight and to stay slim for the rest of your life. If so, what are you willing to do to achieve that goal? What I have discovered is that most people **say** they want to lose weight, but may hesitate when it comes to committing to a lifetime of monitoring. The ex-alcoholic knows that he or she has to practice avoidance of alcohol for the rest of his life. People with life-threatening disorders often have to accept a lifetime of saying no to certain foods or activities. The diabetic knows that he or she cannot eat large quantities of sugar.

What do you know about yourself? You know that left unbridled, you are likely to gain weight eventually reaching an unhealthy proportion. Here I assume you are reading this book because you **do** have a weight problem. The last thing many obese people want to do is to change their eating habits forever. They are happy to take a pill, slurp down diet shakes, and do almost anything, including stapling their stomachs, to avoid the necessity of changing the way they eat real food!

We all know probably at least one person who has tried and tried to lose weight to no avail. The truth is that some people want to keep their problem! To lose weight permanently you must be willing to give up the weight you are carrying and you must be willing to change your eating habits for a lifetime.

For healthy and permanent weight loss results, get off the yo-yo weight loss-weight gain seesaw, and vow to change your eating habits. You will feel so much better. Don't resist, commit.

Pushing on a rope

A friend asked me how I "make" people lose weight. He told me about a fellow who tried every diet imaginable, but who still couldn't lose weight. So, he wanted to know what do I do that's different, how can I make someone lose weight. Unless the person **decides** that it is in their best interest to lose weight no diet in the world will yield permanent results. You must decide that you want to lose weight first. Then you must select the program or diet that suits you. The quick fixes, two-week restriction menus, are unlikely to work for the long term.

What makes this *MAGIC-HAND* Eating Plan your ticket to success is that it is geared for a lifetime, it is easy to use, and most importantly it is extremely flexible. Unlike others, your *MAGIC-HAND* can adapt to almost any situation. Even if you found yourself locked in a room with a carton of chocolate bars for a day, you could still use your *MAGIC-HAND*. That is why you will find success with this Plan. Wherever you go you will always have the tool you need, your hand, with you. Once the program is internalized and you have learned the food groups and how to gauge portion sizes, you will be relying on your **knowledge** of how to eat, not any tables or scales for weighing foods.

What will motivate you to commit to the *MAGIC-HAND* Eating Plan? From observation the two most powerful motivators to lose weight seem to be (1) the experience of having had a heart attack or (2) the anticipation of getting married. Health and vanity-- both are motivating. They are good reasons to lose weight. What's yours? Right now answer this question. Why do you want to lose weight? Will it take a heart attack to move you or are you ready to make the commitment now?

The answer must come from within. The decision to commit to this Eating Plan must be for the rest of your life, every day. The rewards of following this plan will bring you improved health and happiness. I remember what it was like to go shopping for clothes and each time having to try the next larger size. I hated looking at myself in the mirror and it was downright depressing and humiliating not to be able to zip a zipper. Slacks never looked good. I longed for the day I could wear a blouse tucked into the waistband. Now when I look at my clothes I know that I have earned the right to wear them. All of my clothes have stayed in the size 9-10 range (I'm 5ft.8 1/2in.) since reaching my goal in 1981. If for no other reason, I am economically motivated to stay slim. The clothes I have I love, and I want to keep wearing them and looking good. I will do anything to stay this wonderful size, and that's why I stay on the *MAGIC-HAND* Eating Plan. I follow what I preach. Yes, I enjoy looking good. I also enjoy feeling healthy. I have noticed that whenever the calorie-dense foods start to creep into my diet (especially over the December holidays) I truly do not feel as well. It is motivating for me to feel light, to feel healthy, to feel alive, and the closer to the *MAGIC-HAND* I stay, the better is my feeling of well being.

But to get to these rewards, you must decide to eat according to the principles of the *MAGIC-HAND* Eating Plan. If you don't do it, you won't get the reward. Simply put: If you eat all you want, you won't look the way you want. If you want to look the way you want, you can't eat all you want. You would not be reading this book if you were able to control your weight at a desirable level without monitoring your intake. Yes, you **could** exercise more, and that will help, but it probably will still not be enough. You must decide right here and now that you are a person who will commit to keeping your weight under control by monitoring portion-sizes. I have told you how, I have pushed on the rope, but for you to move forward, you must take up the slack on the other side.

It's on the card

Remember the index card we discussed in Practice Point 1? This card is also a motivator. That is why it is so important for you to religiously write down the number on the scale, your weight, every month at your appointed time on the index card. Also, you must tell your buddy. This process stays in place for the rest of your life! If I didn't think you needed constant support, I wouldn't tell you to follow this procedure. But you do, I do, everyone does who has a weight problem. You will be conscious forever that you will have to work to hold the line. Challenges are everywhere. It's not like you can hide food. You **have** to eat to stay well. For you to stay on the program, to stay fit, and to stay slim, it is necessary to stay motivated. When you look at your card and see what you have achieved, you will feel good. When you look at your card and you see that you are maintaining your ideal weight, you will feel terrific. When you look at your card and see that you gained weight, you will then know that you have had a slight misstep and you must spring into action. When you report this to your buddy, you are accountable.

Every month you will get smarter as you study your pattern of fluctuation in weight loss and gain. By keeping notes on all weight gains, you will eventually learn what triggers your eating, or what situations need special attention. You are human, and we all have our ups and downs in life, and often these events are mirrored on the scale. With time and with practice, you will be able to hold your ideal weight.

Invest in yourself for the long haul. You are worthy of a great deal of study and introspection. Being overweight is a complex issue often with more than one cause or underlying factor. If your overeating is psychologically or emotionally charged, expect that it may take longer for you to reach your ideal weight than it would the person who is overweight because of a few bad habits. I know that you are impatient to get the weight off, and you will. But give yourself the time that you need to do it right. As long as you are losing weight every month you are traveling in the right direction. When you seem to stall, it's because your body is fighting to hold on to the weight. Holding the line is also very important. Stay with the program and you will win.

It's your life

Even your best attempts to follow this program will be foiled if you do not truly love yourself. You must be willing to make a commitment to yourself and your health. You must think enough of yourself to believe that you are worth it. Ultimately all the answers to our problems come from within. I cannot make you do anything. Only you can make yourself into the person you want to be. I can offer the blueprint, I can present the example, but you must take the action. The motivation comes from the small voice within that knows and loves you.

When we don't love ourselves, subconsciously we say, " I don't care. I'll eat myself sick." So many people, in fact, do. The major causes of death, chronic diseases, often stem from a lifetime of self-abusive living habits. Is this our cry for help? Is this the way we get attention? Your body is the report card of how much you're hurting, and of how much you care about yourself.

You are responsible, by and large, for your own health within the parameters of predisposing genetic factors. Generally we realize how important our health is when it starts to disappear. People get caught by their bad habits. Look at the cancer patient who smokes. The overweight diabetic. The sedentary high blood pressure patient. These people thought perhaps that they were invulnerable. The truth is that the bad habits we allow into our lives can kill us. Don't you care about the quality of your life? Aren't you good enough to deserve the self-esteem that comes from looking and feeling great?

While I have used the word "magic" to describe my eating plan, both you and I know that what I've given you is a hand trick to make balancing food groups and gauging portion sizes fun and easy. Any diet that takes you away from well-balanced eating is a fad diet. It's not good for the long-term and could even damage your health in the short-term. The most damage that the fad diet does, however, is to keep you from learning the principles of healthy well-balanced eating. It's a shortsighted view of weight loss. It may work for two weeks, but then where are you?

What I'm asking you to do is to change your life habits. Nothing less will do. And in small steps it is a manageable task. What you need is commitment and regular practice. They both go hand in hand. Sometimes you may fight yourself. Remember every day is a new day on the *MAGIC-HAND* Eating Plan. Pick yourself up, start over again. People who quit when they fail will never be successful, but those who get back on track will get to their goals.

Holding on

No matter how long it takes for you to reach your ideal weight, as long as you are on your way with consistent weight loss, stick to the program. The *MAGIC-HAND* Eating Plan relies on your honesty and good sense. You can "cheat" on this program, just as you could on any other. Don't sabotage yourself. The size of your palm is a very specific measure. If you don't believe me, you could measure it with a tape measure. Do not allow yourself to become careless with your "sizing". It's amazing how your palm can grow with loose interpretations.

In your past you may have been caught in a vicious circle. If you've been sedentary, you've probably been so because you were overweight. Conversely, if you are overweight, pounds added because you were sedentary. You may have been uninformed about good nutrition-- not knowing what good, healthy foods to include in your diet. And, of course, some of us learned our bad habits in families where we had to eat what was on our plates whether hungry or not. Don't expect to extinguish every bad habit in a day. You are in training. New habits are developed with practice. Think about how long it took for you to brush your teeth without prompting. It's now a habit in your adult life. You wouldn't feel right without brushing your teeth now. That same thing can happen when you install the *MAGIC-HAND* Eating Plan in your life. You will never be able to look at food the same way again. You will immediately see palm-portions. You will enjoy the results that come from counting.

Two in training

Adele is a spunky woman in her sixties, living alone in a retirement complex. Her problem basically is that she likes to eat, especially peanuts and beer. When she came to me she was on blood pressure medication and carrying 170 pounds on her 5 ft. 1 in. frame. She was unhappy about taking blood pressure pills and wanted to improve her health. Her psychological attitude was wonderful and she had comparatively little stress in her life. But her mental image of herself as a fat lady was devastating. Included in her meditation were affirmations. She said to herself nightly, "I am 160 pounds. It is O.K. for me to weigh less." She began the *MAGIC-HAND* Eating Plan and I asked her to call me when she reached her 160-pound weight sub-goal. Through a combination of meditation, fast walking and using her *MAGIC-HAND* she lost 10 pounds in 3 months. Her next sub-goal is 155 pounds. So far, so good.

Jane is a flight attendant for a major international airline. She has always had a problem keeping her weight under control. Flights take her to Lisbon, Paris, and Cairo, among other cities. She is juggling work stresses, international time changes, and disruptions in her eating patterns every time she flies. Needless to say, she is highly motivated to maintain a slim body weight since flight attendants are expected to present a trim, attractive appearance. She had already experienced just about every quick-loss diet in existence. She was really following the yo-yo method of weight loss. On one regimen she ended in the hospital after trying a liquid protein diet. She was lucky she didn't die. Jane was in fairly good health and her main problem seemed to be her inability to stay with any one diet. She also had a "trick knee" limiting her capability for exercise. She started the *MAGIC-HAND* Eating Plan and was delighted that her measurer, her hand, was always with her. It made eating those pre-packaged flight meals easy to use. She found time to fast-walk almost every day when the weather was good. She had failed to plan ahead with a contingency plan for a cold weather activity so she "lost" three weeks of physical play while she tried to decide what else she could do. It broke the momentum, but with an upcoming wedding to motivate her, she reached her ideal weight in short order. The real challenge came after the wedding when she slipped back to her old eating habits. Then she returned to *MAGIC-HAND* eating proving to herself that she simply cannot hold that line, be in control of her weight, without controlling her portion sizes.

These stories illustrate that we are all human and need to keep the motivation to stay slim to propel us forward. What is **your** reason wanting to stay slim? The best reason you could give me is that you want to feel good about yourself and be the best, healthiest "you" there is. Many women want to become slender in order to attract men or stay fat to keep men away. Some people want to become trim to get a job or to be fat to decrease their chances of being hired. Yet others want to be slim only for their wedding pictures and plan on freely indulging the rest of their married life. Most people are motivated to lose weight for some reason: their doctor has told them, they are getting married, or perhaps they want to look good in a swim suit. People are motivated to fail at losing weight also for some reason: to keep men away, to have a "problem", or perhaps with larger size--gain "authority" to psychologically compensate for the areas in their lives that might be deficient.

Become healthy and slim for yourself, for the pleasure it will bring you, and then nothing can threaten your determination and motivation to win. Although I have consistently emphasized the importance of correct body weight, remember, that as you become more fit, and muscle tissue starts to replace fat tissue, weight gain is possible.

Occasionally take your measurements too. Keep a pair of "target slacks" in your closet and look at yourself. If you start to gain weight and the slacks look better, you'll know the extra weight is due to firmer muscle.

The *MAGIC-HAND* Eating Plan is designed for people who want to lose weight and maintain that loss in a healthy manner. It is also necessary to accept the fact that to effect this change you must permanently install a life style of controlled eating. You may know people who can eat anything and not gain weight, but if you were one of them, you would not be reading this book. So, let's make our pact.

Are we having fun yet?

A sense of humor and losing weight often don't seem to go together. This Plan should be fun. Because weight loss is a multi-faceted issue, many of the answers to why you have this problem must come from within. Think of it as a game. You against excess food. Move the magnets on your *MAGIC-HAND* as if you were winning at checkers or backgammon. Every day you've successfully stayed within or completed all the palm and thumb portions on your *MAGIC-HAND* in all the food groups, you've won. (You know you'll be paying a penalty if you go over the allotted chits.) Every day it's a new game.

Take a look at your hand again. It's a simple little tool that can work for you.

You'll never have to count calories, fat grams or weigh foods again. Remember the slogan: **"My Fingers Count Portions Offering Variety.").** From pinky to thumb you can remember the food groups: **M**ilk & Dairy, **F**ruit, **C**arbohydrate, **P**rotein and **O**ils. These are the players in the game and you must include 3 of each every day. Vegetables are unlimited. A total of 12 finger palm-portions and 3 thumb joints a day!

Now take your left hand and join your thumbs. You have a "**w**" in the middle for water! Four fingers on each hand make 8 glasses a day. Consider yourself in training with the rest of your life to practice. Go for it!

Hand in hand

You want to lose weight. You want to stay at your ideal weight for the rest of your life. Do we know what you want? So, let's begin. I want you to commit to the *MAGIC-HAND* Eating Plan for the next 9 weeks. In that time you will break old habits and learn how to eat properly. I am asking you to devote the next 9 weeks, the next 63 days of your life, to experiencing what healthy eating is like, and to witness your body take new shape. Count the days on your calendar.

After 63 days, you decide if you want to go back to your old way of eating and weight gain. I think you will find that you are happier and healthier at the end of this 9-week period than ever. I want you to prove to yourself that you can do it, and that you can look forward to a lifetime of healthy eating. This investment in a future full of good health and happiness is worth the effort. The initial 9-week period, getting started, is the first big step. To keep yourself motivated study one of the nine workbook focus points each week. If you have friends who want to lose weight, form a group and meet weekly to discuss each focus point. You will find that you learn from others and that their support will keep you going. After you have gone through all nine focus Points, you should be well practiced in the principles of *MAGIC-HAND* eating. At the end of these 9 weeks, ask yourself, "What are the results?" If you have lost weight, and you have found the program liveable make an even deeper commitment to keeping it in place. You now know if it works for you. Can we shake hands on that? If after 63 days of consistently using your *MAGIC-HAND* you have experienced more normal healthy eating, and you have lost weight, and you feel good, vow that you will **commit** to keeping the *MAGIC-HAND* Eating Plan in place for **the rest of your life**.

I believe that your new pattern of eating will be so rewarding that you will be motivated to maintain your results. Consider yourself in training for the Olympics-- but instead this is a training for life. Like any artist or athlete you will always be perfecting your skills and continuing to learn.

If you lose weight, and then go back to your old way of eating, you can expect what? To gain back the weight you lost. Don't do it. Be good to yourself. Love yourself well.

Every day's a new day.
Start.

Go to PRACTICE D9 now.

Now, listen...

the sound of two hands clapping.

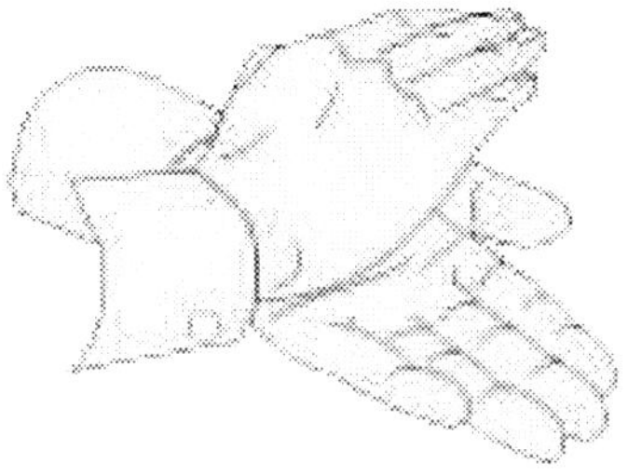

Order Information

This *MAGIC-HAND* Eating Plan course book can be purchased on the *MAGIC-HAND* website: www.*MAGIC-HAND*.org or www.dranne.org

The *MAGIC-HAND* Association operates as a volunteer based, self-sustaining nonprofit organization. Proceeds from the sales of these materials are used to support the website, volunteer activities and provide on-going *MAGIC-HAND* Circle Groups.

Any questions? Send an email to: ask@dranne.org

Appendix A

MAGIC-HAND EQUIVALENT MEASURES

MAGIC-HAND:	**STANDARD:**
For Milk & Dairy, Fruit, Carbohydrates and Proteins:	
1 Palm-portion that's a spooned or soft food =	2-3 Tablespoons
1 Palm-portion that's liquid=	1/4-1/2 cup or 1/3 cup
1 Palm-portion that's rounded & hand held =	1/4-1/2 cup or 1/3 cup
1 Palm-portion that's cut Thumb thick=	1-4 oz.
For Oils & Fats:	
1 Thumb-joint that's solid=	1 teaspoon
1 Thumb-joint that's semi-soft=	1 teaspoon
1 Thumb of oil (if watered down/liquid)=	1 Tablespoon
For Vegetables:	
Unmeasured/ Unlimited	
For Sauces, Gravies, Syrups, Stews, Casseroles, Mixed Beverages, Fast Foods, Exotic Desserts, Preserves, Candy, and Other unidentified foods:	
1 Palm-portion, (sugar/fat laden) liquid, soft or spooned=	2-3 Tablespoons
1 Palm-portion, liquid, rounded, hand-held or cut=	1/4-1/2 cup or 1-4 oz.
1 Thumb (fat/sugar laden) liquid or spooned=	1 Tablespoon
1 Thumb (fat/sugar laden) watered down=	1 Tablespoon
1 Thumb-joint (fat/sugar laden) solid, hard or semi-soft	1 teaspoon

When in doubt:
Each palm-portion ideally should be no more than 100 calories. The default measurement for a palm-portion is 1/3 cup. The less fat in a palm-portion, the fewer will be the calories. The more fiber in a palm-portion, the healthier will be the food. The standard given varies according to the size of your hand.

Appendix B

MAGIC-HAND COOKERY

SOUP, SALAD AND SUCH

FRESH VEGETABLE BORSCH SOUP

1/4 chopped onion
1 cup fresh beets, peeled and diced
2 1/4 cups tomato/vegetable juice
1 T. lemon juice
1 t. fresh parsley, chopped
1/4 cup plain yogurt
1 cup shredded green cabbage
1/2 carrot, shredded
1/2 tomato chopped
1 T. soy sauce (optional)
1/4 t. dill weed

Add onion, beets, cabbage, and carrot to the tomato juice in large saucepan or kettle. Bring to a boil, cover and simmer for 20 minutes. Add tomato, lemon juice and herbs. Simmer for another 15 minutes. When serving, top with a dollop (1 T.) of yogurt.

1 serving= 1/2 Milk chit, Unlimited Vegetable

PITA POCKET MEAL

1 pita bread pocket sandwich
1 slice natural low-fat cheese (2 oz.)
1 t. mayonnaise
1/2 cup alfalfa sprouts
4 oz. fish or chicken
1 t. mustard

Spread mayonnaise and mustard inside pita bread. Stuff with cheese and fish or chicken, and sprouts. Makes 1 serving.

1 serving= 1 Carbohydrate chit, 1 Oil chit, 1 Protein chit

CUCUMBER CHEESE-WITCH

2 palm-size slices sprouted wheat bread
6 thin slices cucumber
1 t. mayonnaise
1/4 cup alfalfa sprouts
1 slice natural swiss cheese (2 oz.)

Spread mayonnaise on bread. Add cheese, cucumber and sprouts on one slice and cover with the other.

1 serving= 2 Carbohydrate chits, 1 Milk chit, 1 Oil chit

SALAD SUPREME

1 palm-portion cheese, poultry or fish
green cabbage
celery
parsley
collard greens
kale
leeks
butter lettuce
mushrooms
green pepper
spinach leaves
watercress
red cabbage
carrots
cucumbers
chard
dandelion greens
mustard greens
romaine lettuce
red and green-leaf lettuce
onions or scallions
radishes
tomatoes
alfalfa sprouts

(I dare you to use them all!) From the above list select your favorite salad ingredients, tear, chop or cut and place in a large salad bowl. Avoid using iceberg lettuce. (It's too boring.) Add chopped broccoli or cauliflower for an interesting touch. Top your serving of greens with a palm-measured portion of sunflower seeds, chopped cheese, poultry or fish. Select a dressing.

1 serving= 1 Protein chit, 1 Oil or 1 Milk chit, Unlimited Vegetable

MANHATTAN BUTTERMILK DRESSING

1 cup buttermilk
1/4 t. dry mustard
1/4 t. lemon juice
4 T. tomato or vegetable juice
1/4 t. garlic powder

Mix all ingredients in a glass container with tight cover. Chill. Shake before serving.
1/4 cup serving= 1 Milk chit

FINE FRENCH DRESSING

6 T. salad/vegetable oil
1 T. rice vinegar
1/4 t. dry mustard
1/4 t. basil
1 clove garlic
2 T. olive oil
1 T. lemon juice
1 t. chopped scallions
pinch of pepper

Place all ingredients in a glass container with tight fitting cover. Shake until thoroughly blended and chill. Allow garlic clove to sit in the bottle.
1 T. serving= 1 Oil chit

BLEU CHEESE DRESSING

2 oz. bleu cheese chunks
1 cup low-fat yogurt
1/4 t. onion powder
2 T. water
2 T. parsley

Stir by hand and chill in refrigerator. Keep in air tight container.
1/4 cup serving= 1 Milk chit

RUSSIAN DRESSING

1 can (8 1/4 oz.) stewed tomatoes plus liquid
3 T. pickle relish
1/2 cup cottage cheese (small curd)
2 T. rice vinegar

Mix together tomatoes and cottage cheese in a blender until smooth. Then, add pickle relish and vinegar and mix. Refrigerate and serve cold.
1/4 cup serving= 1 Milk chit

BREADS AND SPREADS

HEFTY WHEAT PANCAKES

1 cup whole wheat flour
1 egg
1 cup milk
1 t. double-acting baking powder
1 T. honey

Mix together all dry ingredients. Mix egg and honey, then add milk. Combine dry and liquid mixtures. Use a lightly greased pan (or electric skillet set at 360 degrees) and turn over pancakes as soon as edges appear firm. Makes about 8 palm-sized pancakes. (Freeze leftovers and reheat by placing in toaster.)
1 pancake= 1 Carbohydrate chit

RAISIN WHEAT WONDER

2 cups whole wheat/oat flour
1 t. baking powder
1/4 cup wheat germ
1 1/2 cups milk + 1 T. vinegar
3/4 cup raisins
1 T. oats
1 t. baking soda
1/2 t. salt
1/3 cup cooking oil
1/2 cup honey or molasses
1 T. cinnamon

Mix dry ingredients. Add honey to cooking oil, then mix with into soured milk. Mix liquid ingredients with dry ingredients. Let stand uncovered for about 20 minutes. Add raisins and cinnamon. Mix and pour batter into a greased loaf pan (about 9" X 5"). Sprinkle top with oats. Bake for 45 minutes at 400 degrees or until bread is browned and tests dry with a toothpick. Makes 1 loaf.
1 palm-sized, thumb thick serving= 1 Carbohydrate

PEASANT YEAST BREAD

1/4 cup cornmeal
2 packets (1/4 oz.) dry active yeast
1 1/4 cups milk mixed with 1 1/2 T. lemon juice
3/4 cup warm water
1 T. baking powder
5 cups whole wheat/oat flour

Mix warm water with yeast. Cover and let stand for 10 minutes. Add warmed soured milk and baking powder, and stir. Beat in 2 cups of flour for one minute. Cover bowl and let stand for 15 minutes. Slowly beat in remaining flour. Turn out dough on floured board and knead ten minutes or until smooth and elastic. Roll into round or desired shape and place on baking sheet that has been sprinkled with cornmeal. Bake for 30 minutes in preheated 350 degree oven. Makes 2 loaves.
1 palm-size, thumb thick serving= 1 Carbohydrate chit

MOM HOYT'S SPECIAL SPREAD

1 cup cheddar cheese, shredded
1 T. pickle relish
1/4 green pepper, diced
2-3 rolls (cupped-palm size)
1 can (6 oz.) crab meat
1/4 onion, diced
1 t. prepared mustard

Preheat oven to 375 degrees. Mix crab, cheese, relish, onion, pepper and mustard. Slice rolls in half. Spread rounded 1-1 1/2 T. of mixture on each half roll. Bake in oven for 15 minutes or until cheese starts to melt. (Can be served hot or cold.). Makes 2-3 servings.
1 roll serving= 1 Carbohydrate chit, 1 Protein chit

MAIN MEAL ENTREES

BAKED SALMON

2 palm-size salmon filets/steaks
1 T. fresh parsley
1/2 t. dill weed
1/4 fresh cucumber, peeled
1/4 lemon sliced without rind

Place the salmon steak on a sheet of aluminum foil (large enough to wrap the fish). Place very thin cucumber and lemon slices, alternating, on top of fish. Garnish with parsley and dill. Wrap in the aluminum foil and bake for 25 minutes in a preheated 350 degree oven. (Or barbecue in the foil for 20 minutes.) Makes 2 servings.
1 serving= 1 Protein chit

CHICKEN BARBECUE BREAST

4 palm-size chicken breasts or filets
1/8 t. pepper
1/2 t. lemon juice
1/2 cup tomato sauce or salsa
1 clove garlic, minced
1/4 t. prepared mustard
1/4 t. dry mustard

Remove skin from chicken and discard. Prepare the sauce, combining all ingredients and mix by hand. Baste the chicken with sauce and bake in a covered barbecue for 30 minutes. Baste again. Cook for another 15-20 minutes and serve. (Oven alternative: Bake in preheated 350 degree oven for 45 minutes.) Makes 4 servings.
1 serving=1 Protein chit

EGGPLANT PARMESAN

1 medium sized eggplant
1/4 cup cornmeal
1 cup Italian cooking or seasoned tomato sauce
1/4 cup mayonnaise
1 lb. mozzarella cheese

Peel eggplant skin and cut in 1/2 inch slices. Spread mayonnaise thinly on each side of the eggplant slices and pat in cornmeal. Arrange slices on ungreased baking sheet. Bake at 425 degrees for 15 minutes. Then, top each slice with a tablespoon of cooking sauce and 1/2 thumb thick slice mozzarella cheese. Bake at 375 degrees for about 15 minutes or until cheese melts. Heat the remaining cooking sauce and pour over top after serving. Makes 4 servings.

1 serving= 1 Milk chit, 1Oil chit

BRUSSELS SPROUTS SOUFFLE

1/4 cup butter or margarine
1 cup milk
4 egg whites
2 cups cooked Brussels sprouts, chopped
1/4 cup whole wheat or oat flour
4 egg yolks
4 oz. cheddar cheese shredded

Melt butter and blend in the flour. Add milk and cook until mixture thickens, stirring constantly for white sauce. Remove from heat. Beat egg yolks until thick and lemon-colored. Slowly blend the egg yolks into the white sauce and stir rapidly. Add in shredded cheese, finely chopped Brussels sprouts. Beat egg whites until stiff, but not dry; fold into mixture. Pour into an ungreased 2-quart souffle dish. Bake in moderate oven, 350 degrees, for 40 minutes or until knife inserted comes our clean. Makes 4 servings.

1 serving or 2 cupped palms= 1 Protein chit, 1 Milk chit

WHITE SAUCE

1 t. butter or margarine
1/2 cup milk (at least 2% fat)
1 T. enriched white flour
(optional: 1 T. mixed carrots and peas)

Melt butter in saucepan. Remove from heat and mix in four. Slowly add milk over heat and bring to slow boil for about one minute, mixing constantly until thickened. (Add carrots and peas.) Serve immediately. Makes 1 serving.

1 serving= 1 Milk chit, 1 Oil chit

MOTHER'S VEGETABLE COMBINATION DISH

4 cups vegetables in season (broccoli, squash, carrots, etc.)
1/2 cup natural cheddar cheese, shredded
1/2 cup brown rice

Cook brown rice and let stand. Steam vegetables for about 15 minutes until just tender. Place the hot vegetables in the center of a large serving place and top with the shredded cheese. While cheese is melting ring the vegetables with rice. Serve immediately. Makes 2 servings.

1 serving= 1 Carbohydrate chit, 1 Milk chit

SHEPHERD'S POT LUCK

1/2 cup leftover meat
1 can V-8 juice/ tomato juice
pepper, garlic to taste
2 palm-size potatoes mashed
2 cups assorted vegetables plus onion
1/4 cup milk
1 t. Worcestershire sauce
paprika

Preheat oven to 375 degrees. In 1 1/2 quart casserole dish combine meat, vegetables, onion, pepper and Worcestershire sauce. Pat down evenly in dish. Make mashed potatoes by cooking, mashing and mixing with 2 t. butter and 1/4 cup milk. Place tablespoons of mashed potatoes on top and spread to cover mixture. Sprinkle with paprika. Bake 40 minutes or until golden brown and bubbly. Makes 2 servings.

1 serving= 1 Protein chit, 1 Carbohydrate chit, 1 Oil chit

MEATLESS MOUSSAKA

1/2 onion, chopped
1/4 t. pepper
1 can (16 oz.) tomatoes, drained
1 large eggplant, long shape
1/2 cup milk
1 t. cooking oil
1 T. parsley
1/4 t. nutmeg
1/4 cup seasoned tomato sauce
4 eggs
1 cup mozzarella cheese, grated

Peel and thinly slice eggplant. Put half of slices on bottom of lightly greased 2-quart casserole. Brown the onion in oil and add to mixture of tomatoes, tomato sauce, milk, parsley, pepper and nutmeg. Pour mixture over eggplant slices. Place remaining eggplant slices on top. Cover and bake for 30 minutes in a 375 degree oven. Beat the eggs and stir into warm, not hot casserole. Top with cheese and bake uncovered for 15 minutes or more. Makes 4 servings.
1 serving= 1 Protein chit, 1 Milk chit

CHILI A LA LOUISE

2 cups red kidney beans
1 garlic clove, chopped
1 bay leaf
1 t. cooking oil
3/4 cup bean liquid
1/4 t. red cayenne pepper
1 cup celery chopped
1 onion, chopped
1 sprig parsley
1/4 t. salt
1/4 green pepper, chopped
1 t. chili powder
4 tomatoes, chopped

Rinse beans and let stand overnight in a pot filled with 4 cups of water. Add 1/4 onion, garlic, parsley, bay leaf and salt to the soaking water, cover and simmer 1 hour until the beans are tender. Drain the solids from the liquid, retaining 3/4 cup bean liquid. Remove bay leaf and parsley sprig. Saute 1/2 onion and green pepper in cooking oil until slightly browned. Remove from heat. Add back bean liquid; then add chili powder, red pepper, chopped tomatoes and celery. Stir in kidney beans. Simmer mixture over low heat for at least 45 minutes. Makes 4 servings.
1 serving= 1 Protein chit

BAKED POTATO PROUD

1 cupped palm Russet potato
1 T. chives
2 T. sour cream or yogurt
dash pepper

Bake potato in 425 degree oven for about 45 minutes. Cut an "X" across the top and puff up the potato by pushing the sides towards the center. Create an indention in the middle and fill with sour cream or yogurt and chives, then add pepper. Makes 1 serving.
1 serving= 1 Carbohydrate chit, 1 Milk chit

TURKEY BREAST BAKE

4 oz. turkey breast slices
2 t. prepared mustard
dash pepper
1/4 cup corn meal
2 oz. mozzarella cheese

Lightly spread mustard on turkey slices and pat in corn meal. Place on cooking sheet and bake in preheated 450 degree oven for 10 minutes. Top with mozzarella cheese and a dash of pepper. Return to oven for another 5 minutes or until cheese is melted. Makes 1 serving.
1 serving= 1 Protein chit, 1 Milk chit

DESSERTS

BLUEBERRY COBBLER

1 cup whole wheat/oat flour
1/4 t. salt
1 t. lemon juice
1/4 cup butter or margarine, soft
1/2 cup milk
1 1/2 t. baking powder
12 oz. blueberries
1/2 cup water
1 egg slightly beaten
1 1/2 t. vanilla

Mix flour, baking powder and salt. Mix egg, milk and vanilla, then add butter. Combine dry and liquid ingredients slowly mixing and beating them well. Pour blueberries, water and lemon juice mixture in bottom of 1 1/2 greased quart casserole. Spoon batter over top. Bake for 30 minutes in preheated 375 degree oven. Makes 4 servings.

1 serving or 2 cupped palms= 1 Fruit chit, 1 Carbohydrate chit

DEBBIE'S DELIGHT COOKIES

1 1/2 cups whole wheat/oat flour
1 3/4 cups old fashioned oats
1/2 t. salt
1/2 cup honey/brown sugar
1 t. vanilla
1/2 cup bran
1/2 t. baking soda
1/4 cup cooking oil
1 egg ,well beaten
1/2 cup chopped walnuts
1 cup mashed over-ripe banana (or applesauce, cooked squash, cooked pumpkin)
1/2 cup raisins

Mix all dry ingredients. Then add all mixed liquids and include banana, walnuts and raisins. Place batter in rounded tablespoons on greased cookie sheet. Bake for 15 minutes in 350 degree oven. Makes about 5 dozen cookies (textured and crunchy).

2 cookies= 1 Carbohydrate chit

COCO MOUSSE

1 envelope (1T.) unflavored gelatin
2 T. Hershey's cocoa (unsweetened)
1 t. vanilla extract
1 can (13 oz.)evaporated skimmed milk
1 T. dark brown sugar
(optional: 1/4 t. mint extract)

Mix cocoa and sugar in 1/4 cup milk until blended. In a medium saucepan gradually sprinkle gelatin over remainder of milk, cooking over low heat and stirring until gelatin is dissolved. Add cocoa mixture and stir until blended. Pour the mixture into a 1 1/2 quart mixing bowl and set aside to cool (or place in refrigerator about 15 minutes). Add vanilla. (Add mint.) Beat at high speed with electric mixer until thick and foamy. Place in covered container and refrigerate until firm. (Or store in freezer. Allow 20 minutes to defrost.) Makes 4 servings.

1 serving= 1 Milk chit

FRUIT AND CHEESE BOARD

sliced fresh pineapple
sliced red delicious apples
farmer's cheese
Thompson seedless grapes
low-fat cheddar cheese

Arrange on a platter board, slice of apple and pineapple. Accent with small bunches of grapes. Put cheese slices to one side and eat in combination with fruit.

1 cupped-palm serving= 1 Fruit chit

1 palm-size, thumb thick cheese or 2 oz.= 1 Milk chit

Appendix C
SEEING FINGERS

These lists give you a good idea of what foods fall into various food group categories. Some foods can be counted under more than one food group. Note that even though botanically a tomato is a fruit, we count it as a Vegetable.

MILK & DAIRY PRODUCTS

Buttermilk
Camembert
Cheddar
Cottage cheese
Cream cheese/Neufchatel
Farmer's cheese
Hoop cheese
Ice cream/Ice milk
Milk: whole, 2%, skim
Parmesan
Pudding/custard
Swiss cheese
Whipped cream
Yogurt

If you are allergic to MILK & DAIRY PRODUCTS, here are some substitutes high in calcium:

Palm-portions *-high calcium*
Almonds
Canned mackerel
Canned salmon
Canned sardines
Chickpeas (garbanzo beans)
Dried figs
Filberts
Fortified bread
Oats, Oatmeal
Pistachio nuts
Red or white pinto beans
Sesame seeds
Tofu

Unlimited *-high calcium*
Beets
Broccoli
Collard greens
Kale
Mustard greens
Okra
Parsley
Raw collard greens
Spinach
Turnip greens

FRUIT & FRUIT JUICES

Apples
Apricots
Avocado
Bananas
Berries
Cantaloupe
Cherries
Dates
Figs
Fruit pies
Grapefruit
Grapes
Kiwi fruit
Lemons and limes
Mandarins
Mangos
Melons
Nectarines
Olives
Oranges
Papayas
Peaches
Pears
Persimmons
Pineapple
Plums
Prunes
Raisins
Rhubarb (sweetened)
Strawberries
Tangerine

CARBOHYDRATES & STARCHY VEGETABLES

Bagels
Barley
Beans: black, kidney, lima, navy, pinto
Biscuits
Bran
Breads
Buckwheat
Cakes
Cereals
Cookies
Corn
Crackers
Croissants
Croutons
Danish pastry
Doughnuts
Edame
English muffins
Grits
Ice cream cone
Jello
Lentils
Millet
Muffins
Oatmeal
Pancakes, waffles
Parsnips
Pasta
Peas
Pita
Popcorn
Potato chips
Potatoes
Pretzels
Pumpkin
Rice, rice cakes
Rolls
Rye
Snow peas
Squash: winter, acorn, butternut
Stuffing (bread-base)
Sweet potatoes
Tortillas
Wheat, wheat germ

PROTEIN SOURCES

Almonds
Beef
Black beans
Cheese
Chicken
Cold cuts
Duck
Eggs
Filberts
Fish: bass, cod, flounder, halibut, herring, salmon, sardines, shark, snapper, swordfish trout, tuna, yellowtail, etc.
Game
Goose
Green peas
Kidney beans
Lamb
Lentils
Lima beans
Liver
Lox/Smoked fish
Macadamia nuts
Navy beans
Organ meats
Peanuts
Pecans
Pinto beans
Pork
Pumpkin seeds
Sausages/ frankfurters
Shellfish: calamari, clams, crab, crayfish, lobster, mussels, octopus, oysters, scallops, shrimp, squid, etc.
Soy
Sunflower seeds
Tofu
Turkey
Veal
Walnuts
Yogurt

OILS & FATS

(AND CONCENTRATED SUGARS)

Barbeque sauce
Butter/Margarine
Caramel
Chocolate fudge
Coconut oil
Gravy (oil-base)
Hard candy/chocolates
Ice cream syrup
Jams and jellies, preserves
Mayonnaise
Nut and seed butters
Pancake/maple syrup
Peanut butter
Salad dressing
Sweet sauces, toppings, etc.
Vegetable oils

VEGETABLES & HERBS

Artichokes
Asparagus
Beets
Broccoli
Brussels Sprouts
Cabbage
Carrots
Cauliflower
Celery
Chard
Cilantro
Cucumbers
Eggplant
Endive
Escarole
Fennel
Garlic
Green, red chilies
Green, yellow string beans
Herbs, all
Horseradish
Jicama
Kale
Ketchup
Leeks
Mushrooms
Mustard
Okra
Onions
Peppers
Pickles
Radishes
Rhubarb (raw)
Rutabaga
Salad greens
Salsa/Picante
Sauerkraut
Scallions
Spices
Spinach
Sprouts, bamboo shoots
Squash: summer, spaghetti, chayote
Sun chokes
Tomatoes
Turnips
Vegetable juices
Water chestnuts
Watercress
Zucchini

MAGIC-HAND®

Eating Plan

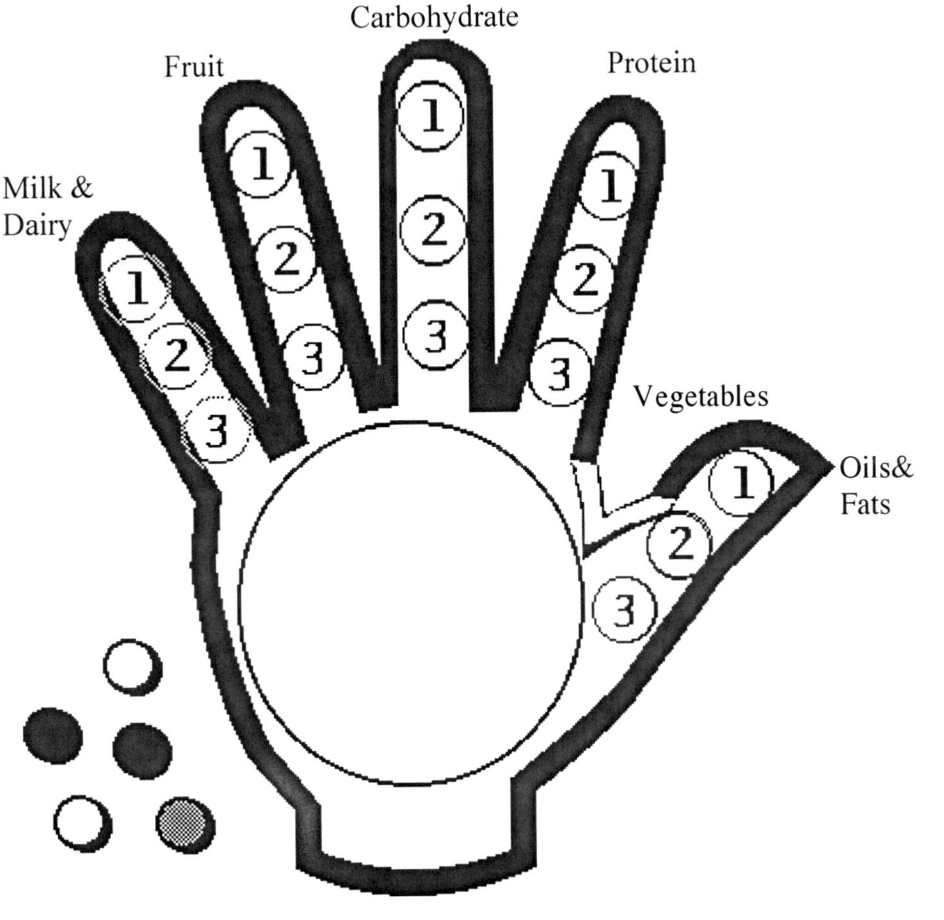

PRACTICE

Introduction

Our mission is to promote healthy well-balanced eating for weight control and to make it easy and fun. Also, to provide on-going support groups in every neighborhood. And to give you a way to keep your weight under control that is flexible and livable for a lifetime.
Most people need support when changing habits and this book is the start-point. To stay motivated we strongly recommend that you participate in a *MAGIC-HAND* sponsored Circle Group. If a *MAGIC-HAND* Eating Plan support circle does not already exist in your area, you may need to establish your own. See Appendix F for details.

The purpose of the *MAGIC-HAND* PRACTICE is to provide guidelines and useful exercises to be completed sometimes in the privacy of your own company or in a Circle Group setting. By writing down your answers you can help yourself become clear about where you stand on psychological, physical and practical issues. You are forced to think about your lifestyle and what is good for you. Make sure to write down your answers to the questions posed since this act makes your words in thought definite.

You can't help someone who doesn't want to help himself.
Guidance for the changes you are willing to make. Practice for life.

*M*easure

M1

● Point 1

Getting your numbers

Let's establish your health baseline according to some physical and physiological measurements. Plan to update and review these measures every year as part of your own physical evaluation. As you lose weight you will see these measures improve.

Do this at home: the 'Mirror Test'

(This may take courage, but do it anyway.) Stand in front of a full-length mirror without any clothes and take a good look. Point your toes forward and observe your body shape. Imagine a line going lengthwise through the center of your body. Are you lopsided? Standing straight? Now turn sideways. Squeeze your buttocks and pull in your "stomach" abdominal muscles.

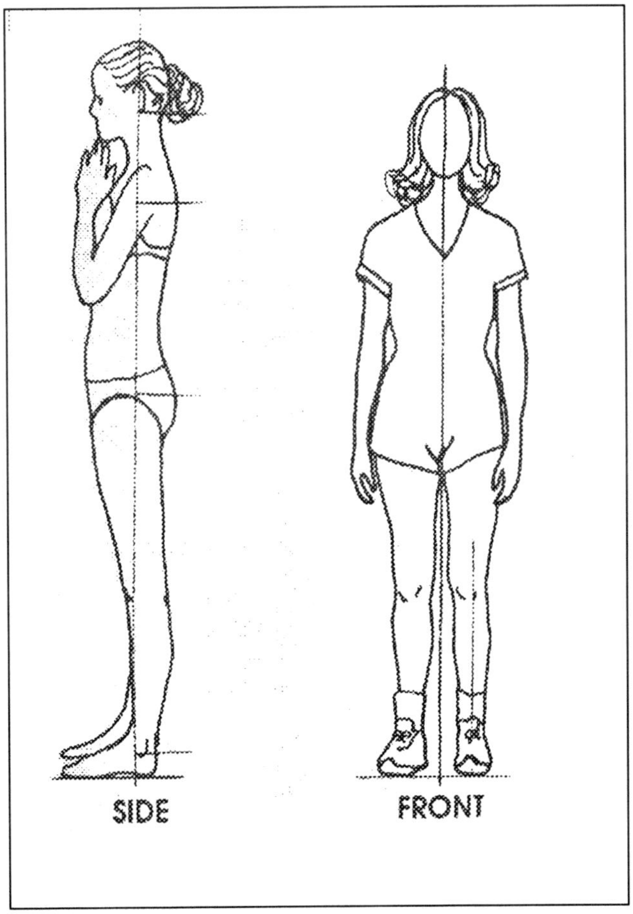

Do this now: While seated, place your hands on your mid-section and find your abdominal muscles. Can you locate them?
While exhaling, try to pull them in. Breathe out and tighten your abdominals.

Notice any difference? Any thoughts about your body?

____

Homework Special Assignment: Now, take the "pulse test". This is an indicator of your cardiovascular health. While you are lying in bed-- before you arise in the morning-- find your pulse by placing your middle fingers on the side of the neck just under your jawbone. Using the second hand on your watch or clock, count the number of heartbeats you feel in 15 seconds. Then multiply this number by 4 to get the number of heartbeats in a minute (60 seconds). Repeat this procedure until you get a consistent number. If your pulse rate is over 80 beats per minute you are out of condition!
15 second pulse rate is: _____X 4 =_______ beats per minute.

A field trip! Your Medical records: If you have results from a recent blood test or physical exam, insert this information in the Summary Table given below. If you have not been tested within the last two years, it's time! Do you know your blood pressure?
A healthy reading is near 120/80. Anything over 140 is considered "high".

If you haven't already done so, get a blood test to include your personal health "markers". Look for changes in your own baseline blood test values to indicate changes in your health status. Although influenced by genetics and your thyroid, divide your cholesterol value by the HDL (High-Density-Lipoproteins) to get the heart risk-ratio. If the answer is above 4.5 you may be at risk for heart disease. A triglyceride value above 165 is considered "high". Remember that blood test results and blood pressures vary so do not rush into medicating if lifestyle change might work first. Retesting is prudent. Generally, you will benefit from weight reduction and exercise. You are taking a good step in the direction towards bettering test results and improving your health.

Below is a sample table to record your starting health benchmarks.
Fill in as much information as you can now on this summary table or create your own.

SUMMARY TABLE

TEST	VALUE	DATE
(insert tests important to me)		
WEIGHT	__________	_______
RESTING PULSE	__________	_______
BLOOD PRESSURE	__________	_______
CHOL/HDL RATIO	__________	_______
TRIGLYCERIDES	__________	_______
____________________	__________	_______
____________________	__________	_______
____________________		

Update this table every year. Enter next exam date: __________

The right range numbers

(If you are sure and you already know your ideal weight you can skip this section.)

Your weight is the number that registers on the scale. The goal is to maintain an ideal weight-- to see that number register as the best weight for your body design. If you are not sure what the best or ideal healthy weight is for yourself, here is a simple formula you can use:

For women, start with 100 lbs. for five feet of height. For every inch over five feet add 5 pounds. For example, if you are 5 feet 4 inches in height, you should weigh 100 lbs. + 20 lbs.= 120 pounds assuming an average or medium frame body build.

For men, start with 106 lbs. for five feet of height. For every inch over five feet add 6 pounds. Making this more complicated, let's say you are a 6' 3 1/2" man, then your ideal weight according to this formula, given a medium frame, would be 106 + (15.5 in. X 6 lbs.) or 93 = 199 pounds. But, assuming you are large boned, you would then add 10%, for an "ideal weight" of (199 + 19.9) = 218.9 or, rounding off, 219 pounds.

Here is a quick and easy way to determine if you are "small-boned" or "large-boned". Measure the circumference of your non-dominant wrist at its smallest part by wrapping the thumb and middle finger of the other hand around it.

You are small-boned if your thumb and middle finger overlap. You are large-boned if the fingers don't touch. If the fingers just touch you are medium framed.

If you are small-boned subtract 10% from your answer. If you are large-boned add 10% to your answer. (Remember these estimates are approximate and by no means the last word on what you should weigh. Muscle tissue weighs more than fat tissue so if you are very muscular this estimate might be low and conversely, if you have a lot of fat tissue and little muscle, this estimate might be too high.)

Guideline to my "ideal" weight:
100 lbs. + ________ = ________ (add/subtract 10%)=________
106 lbs. + ________ = ________ (add/subtract 10%)=________
My "ideal" weight according to this formula is: ____________

I agree with this? YES or NO

Why?

____

____

Make sure you do this now!
The "ideal" weight I have set for myself is: ____________

My "ideal weight range" is established by subtracting and adding two pounds to my "ideal" weight. Write down your ideal weight range from low to high with the ideal weight in the middle. Circle or underline your ideal weight.

My Ideal Weight Range is :________ ________ ________
Low -2 Ideal +2 High

My present weight is: ____________ Date: ____________

Every **month** I will report my weight to my buddy. My buddy is: ____________________

Every **month** I will record my weight on a 3 X 5 index card.
The date I have chosen as my monthly recording date is: ____________________
(If you don't have an Index Card, use the one on the bottom of this page.)

For Circle Group Discussion:
How can I best take care of my health? (Answer this question for yourself first.)____________________

____

____

____

____

How healthy am I? What health benefit will I get from losing weight? (In a few sentences answer these questions for yourself first.)

____

____

____

____

Find an index card or use the one below. Tape the card inside your bath medicine cabinet or a closet door.
Index card cut-out: Write your name and weight information on the top line of the card.

On the top line: (your name) -2 (Ideal Weight) +2 Year:

Date (Day)	Weight	Note:

Apportion

A2

● Point 2

Getting to know FINGER FOODS

What foods do I really like to eat? Write down a list of your favorite foods that you usually like to eat. After the food indicate with an "X" whether or not it is a "trigger" food for you, that is, once you have one you can't stop having another.

From your list of favorite foods identify where it belongs in a food group. Some foods may be a combination of different foods (like pizza) so decide how you might wish to categorize the food. In this case, for example, you could call it a "Carbohydrate" or a "Milk" or even a "Protein". You could list it under one or all three. In actual practice you will be counting your palm-size portion in one of these food groups, but when foods are in combination there is some flexibility.

Write down all the foods that would fall in the "**Milk and Dairy**" food group:

______________________ ______________________

______________________ ______________________

______________________ ______________________

______________________ ______________________

Write down all the foods from your list that fall under the "**Fruit**" food group category:

______________________ ______________________

______________________ ______________________

______________________ ______________________

______________________ ______________________

Write down all the foods from your list that fall under the "**Carbohydrate**" food group:

______________________ ______________________

______________________ ______________________

______________________ ______________________

______________________ ______________________

Write down all the foods from your list that fall under the "**Protein**" food group:

______________________ ______________________

______________________ ______________________

______________________ ______________________

______________________ ______________________

Write down all the foods from your list that fall under the "**Oils and Fats**" food group:

______________________ ______________________

______________________ ______________________

______________________ ______________________

______________________ ______________________

Write down all the foods that fall under the (*non-starchy*) **"Vegetable"** food group: and/or are "Unlimited" (tea, etc.):

____________________________ ____________________________

____________________________ ____________________________

____________________________ ____________________________

____________________________ ____________________________

Did you have at least one favorite food that was in each of the six food groups? If not, you might want to take another look at the Seeing Fingers Appendix C at the end of the *MAGIC-HAND* MANUAL section. Try to find the foods in each food group that you like and add them to the food group lists above to create your own special menus.

Designing your daily menu

To practice eating the *MAGIC-HAND* way, design your own menu. Custom tailor each day so that you include foods from each of the food groups and calculate the number of palm-portion chits. Use the foods you previously listed in each of the food groups to create a menu that you'll enjoy eating. If you are better at following a structured menu plan, repeat this process for the next 7 days. Then make believe that you are on a "diet"-- and this is what you have to eat. Thereafter you are the master who can create and follow well-balanced menus. Using your palm-portions you will keep your weight under control long-term. Go for it!

My Menu

Meal	Food Group Item	Palm/thumb portion
Breakfast (Time)		
Snack:		
Lunch: (Time)		
Snack:		
Dinner: (Time)		

Total Number of Palm-portions:______ **Total Number** of Thumb-portions:______

For Circle Group discussion:
What foods do I really like to eat? How would I measure the portion-size? In what food group or groups does it belong?

Good

Point 3

How much should I exercise?

You must determine for yourself the physical play activities you want to pursue. The objective is to find pleasure or joy in what you select.

Before we discuss what is feasible, let's take a look at a number of physical play activities. Without thinking of the exercise benefits of any these activities, go through the list and check the ones that you "like" or for some reason, appeal to you. This list includes over fifty activities enjoyable to a great many people. Of course, there are more, so add any others that you might like as well. From this list select those activities that excite you. Don't concern yourself now with any limitations you may have in pursuing the activity. (I know if you live in Florida you won't be going skiing every day.) Never mind. Simply go through the list and quickly place a check mark next to your favorite activities or those you'd like to do.

__Fast/race walking	__Weight lifting	__Tap dancing	__Water skiing
__Yoga	__Square dancing	__Archery	__Badminton
__Baseball/Softball	__Basketball	__Back-packing	__Bicycling
__Bowling	__Boxing/Wrestling	__Calisthenics	__Canoeing
__Cross-country ski	__Mtn. climbing	__Diving/board	__Ballet
__Aerobic dancing	__Ballroom dancing	__Fencing	__Flexibility exercises
__Football/touch	__Gardening	__Handball	__Snowshoeing
__Squash	__Tennis	__Hiking	__Trampoline/mini
__Ice/figure skating	__Horseback riding	__Hockey field/ice	__Golf
__Gymnastics	__Judo/karate	__Aikido/T'ai chi	__Lacrosse
__Paddle ball	__Ping pong	__Cricket	__Racquetball
__Rugby	__Running	__Jogging/course	__Rope skipping
__Sailing/yachting	__Skateboard	__Scuba/skin diving	__Skiing/downhill
__Roller skating	__Soccer	__Swimming	__Shuffleboard
__Rowing	__Bocce ball	__Ballroom dance	__Surfing board/wind
__Volleyball	__Other............	__................	__.................

Many activities are only enjoyable if the weather is good, but we can plan around that. Let's analyze and plan a physical play program designed especially for you and your life circumstances. This will become the overall picture of your physical play program.

Start to fill in the table below for all the activities you checked. (If you have more than nine, try to narrow your list or if you want to keep them, get another sheet of paper.) Imagine yourself participating in each of the activities selected and decide what factors contribute to your joy. Write down the seasons (Su, F, W, S) appropriate to the enjoyment of the activity. Look at your list and decide what physical play activities are fun and **when**. Again, think back to your childhood. If basketball is on your list, when did you play? In the spring? In the rain? Outdoors or indoors? Are there some activities that you enjoy in every season and in all types of weather?

My Physical Play Program

ACTIVITY	SEASON Su,F,W,S	INDOORS OUTDOORS	GROUP? Partner?	EQUIPMENT needed?	CONVENIENT	WEATHER factor?
1.						
2.						
3.						
4.						
5.						
6.						
7.						
8.						
9.						

Now analyze your list and select the activities that appear to be reasonable choices for your regular participation. Consider your present situation. Do you live in the country or the city? What activities on your list could become "regular, frequent" activities and what activities on your list are only "occasionally" possible?

Your exercise prescription

You need to get started. And the time is now. What is the season now? Let's look at your list again. Select a favorite activity that would be appropriate for this season. Of all the convenient, fun, possible physical play activities on your list, which one will you select to start?

Exercise Prescription

Season: ______________________________

Main play activity:______________________________

Alternatives/Back-up:______________________________

____

Place: ______________________________

How often: ______________________________

What length of time: ______________________________

For Circle Group participation:
Knowing how to walk properly and hold your body is a basic first step to any physical activity. With someone seated across the room watching you, walk five steps forward. Are your feet straight? Do you walk as if on a straight line or are your toes pointing out or in? Is your body aligned?

For Circle Group discussion:
Do you want to set aside a specific amount of time (at least 20 minutes) during the day for physical play or would you rather accumulate times of activity (at least 30 minutes) throughout the day. What would be easier for you?

____

Describe, if you can, the routine in your life. Do you go to work Monday through Friday? Are you at home most of the time? Are you traveling a lot? Where will you get your 20 minutes every other day or your accumulated 30 minutes of physical play?

____

____

____

____

____

____

Do you have any obstacles right now to starting your physical activity? If so, what are they? How can they be overcome?

*I*nner

● Point 4

How do my mind and body interact?

Some part of you must decide that you deserve to become the person you want to be both physically and psychologically. Are you fighting yourself? Your feelings may be controlling your eating behavior. We will explore some of those feelings in this Practice section. It is time for you to take charge of those emotions.

Is there something about my body that I do not like? If so, what?

Would losing weight make it better?

What is it about my body that I do like?

Try to visualize your body at your ideal weight. See this as your achievable goal. Whenever you think about your body or look at yourself in the mirror see yourself at your ideal weight or if you have a lot of weight to lose, just see yourself with five pounds less.

A mental exercise

Visualize yourself as you are right now. Keep taking off five pounds until you reach your ideal weight. Every time you take off five pounds ask yourself, "How do I feel?" Was that weight serving any purpose? If not, release that fat visually. Let it go. Say to yourself: "I am on my way to my ideal weight." And be happy. Put a smile on your face. Know that with the *MAGIC-HAND* you can achieve and maintain your ideal weight goal for a lifetime.

Very important

Your feelings are very important and will either assist you or sabotage you as you get closer to your ideal weight. Not only must you stay with Dr. Anne's *MAGIC-HAND* Eating Plan, but you must also become keenly aware of the times when you overeat or binge or simply stuff yourself. Do not consider these events as failures-- they are learning opportunities crucial to your eventual success! You might wish to keep a journal and record the date, precipitating event, your feelings, your reaction, and upon reflection, what you could do other than eating to handle your emotions.

Take charge

If you gain weight during a month, there is a reason why. Whenever you record an increase in weight from the previous month on your index card, describe in one or two words on the same line the event or circumstance that you feel is responsible under the heading "Note". Then determine what you could do differently or if there is an emotional factor that deserves your introspection. For example, you might have gained weight because of not counting palm-portions at your sister's birthday party, or because of an emotional upset from an ex-spouse's visit, or simply from counting ice cream in your Milk food group too many times. Determine how you will handle these situations and your use of food the next time to prevent weight gain. If you notice that every time your ex-spouse visits you gain weight because of an eating binge try to identify the feeling (anger?) and attempt either through your own self-talk or with a counselor to resolve the hurt. Get in control.

Overeating style

How would you describe your weight-gain eating style?

Are you a High Intake Appestat eater?________________

Are you a Food Trigger Binger?________________________

Are you a Stuffing Feelings Eater?___________________

A combination?______________________________________

Think back to a time when you simply ate too much, or had a binge eating episode, or just kept stuffing yourself with food. Can you remember what happened or how you were feeling? Describe.

____

____

____

Now take this feeling(s) and think of another action you could take (besides eating) that would make you feel better or could help you to release the emotion? Complete the sentence:

When I am feeling_____________ I could ____.

When I am feeling_____________ I could____.

When I am feeling_____________ I could____.

When I am feeling_____________ I could____.

For Circle Group discussion:
Try to identify the mood you are in right now. Say "I'm feeling______________." Someone in the group volunteer to tell a short funny story and no matter how funny or unfunny it is, everyone must laugh with a "ho,ho,ho". Go ahead.

Now, how are you feeling? Did your mood change? Do you have the power to change how you're feeling?

___

Control

● Point 5

How can I find the time to stay healthy?

Let's look at a day in your life. Using the clock diagram below describe your own "typical" day, from the time you get up in the morning until the time you go to bed in the evening. (Pick a day during the week if you're employed outside the home.) Identify blocks of time by drawing a line from the center of the clock to the outside perimeter. Inside each wedge-shaped block of time write in the activity that occurs in that time period for your "typical" day.

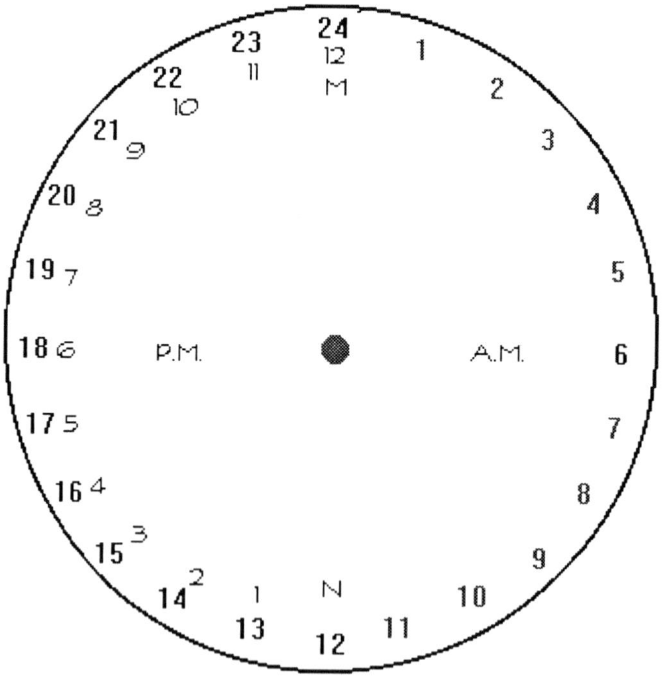

Right now, does your day include some time for eating regular meals, for physical play or exercise, and for meditation?

If not, let's find some time to include these activities. Study your day and determine when you might include the practices you need to stay healthy. For example, you could include physical exercise before breakfast in the morning, perhaps before lunch, before dinner or before bedtime. Could you meditate after lunch or after dinner or before bedtime? Where are your opportunities for exercise or physical play? When could you take 20 minutes for meditation? To feel good, how many hours of sleep do you require?

Redraw your clock diagram so that these health practices are included on a regular basis.

- (1) First draw in the times that you will spend eating meals
- (2) then the time(s) that you will exercise, and lastly
- (3) a time for meditation
- After these priorities, add the other activities that normally consume your day.

Complete this diagram including the appropriate physical play activity you have selected for this season.

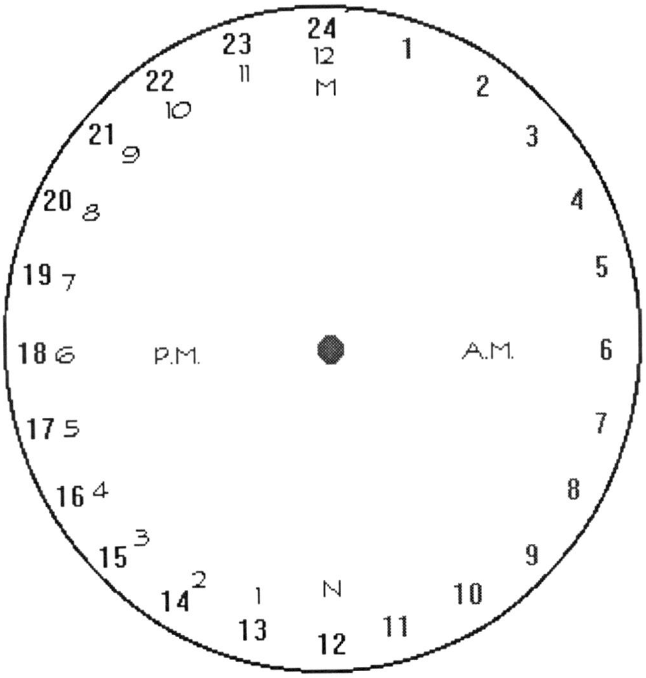

For Circle Group discussion:
Are others in my life robbing me of time? If so, what could I do differently to put my needs first? State one concrete action.

____

____

____

At present do I make time to eat regular meals?

____

____

At present do I make time to meditate or reflect quietly for about 20 minutes each day?

____

____

At present do I make time for a regular physical play exercise activity?

____

____

What would I have to do to get the time I need to stay healthy? State one concrete action you could take immediately to free twenty minutes in your day.

____

____

____

Have I scheduled a regular time each month for entering my weight on my index-card?

____

Sept 7

*H*old

● Point 6

Four MUSTS

After you have reached your ideal weight, you can start the challenging process of learning how to maintain that weight. Remember your weight range. If ever you go two pounds over your ideal weight, you **MUST** return to strictly adhering to the food groups and portion controls of the *MAGIC-HAND* Eating Plan.

There are two basic approaches to loosening the restrictions of the *MAGIC-HAND* for maintaining your ideal weight. One is simply to start bringing back into your diet some of the foods you enjoy that you know are very calorie-dense. You can bring these foods back in palm-portions while still staying on the *MAGIC-HAND* Eating Plan. Another approach is to use the *MAGIC-HAND* only on certain days of the week and not on others. You will discover for yourself how far you can deviate without gaining weight through a process of trial and error. And you **MUST** vow to return strictly to the rules of the *MAGIC-HAND* Eating Plan if through your experimentation you start to gain weight. You **MUST** stay very conscious of eating in palm-portions. This is a forever diet. Remember, your old ways of eating resulted in disaster! Whatever you do-- do not think you're on holiday because you've achieved your goal and interpret that accomplishment as a signal that you can now return to your old eating habits. You **MUST** keep the *MAGIC-HAND* Eating Plan in place. Never let it go entirely.

Consider for a moment if there are any favorite foods you do not eat in order to lose weight. List the foods in the left column.

If you were to start eating them again in what food group category would they belong? For each food you listed, describe how you could serve that food in a palm/thumb-portion serving.

Favorite Food	**Food Group**	**Palm/thumb-portion**

What food group(s) do I like the most or want to eat most? ____________________

____

What food group(s) do I like the least or have difficulty getting into my diet?

____

Could I meet the nutritional benefit of the food group(s) I don't like in some other way? How? ____

____

____

Could I "trade-in" some chits from a food group I don't like to a food group I do like without gaining weight? ____

____

Each person can learn to modify the *MAGIC-HAND* Eating Plan so that it is tailored to his or her specific likes and dislikes. For example, you can trade the chits in one food group to another, but the more you deviate from the balanced principles of *MAGIC-HAND* eating, the less healthy the diet is likely to become. Nevertheless there is a definite convenience to maintaining your weight on the Plan when you can trade your chits. Ultimately it makes the *MAGIC-HAND* Eating Plan very livable and flexible. It also means that you can eat what everyone else is eating and what you like to eat, but always in moderation.

At your ideal weight (or to maintain your weight), how much do you think you can deviate from *MAGIC-HAND* eating without gaining weight? What could you permit?

____

____

For Circle Group discussion:

Did you discover any ways to "stretch" your favorite foods with vegetables? If so, how?

____

____

Are there any food preparation tricks you use to make healthful desserts?

____

____

What has been the most challenging problem for you to overcome with food preparation?

____

____

____

Food Preparation Ideas:

Adapt

● Point 7

Eating challenges

How can I handle eating away from home? Fortunately you can plan ahead to meet the challenges of restaurant dining, house parties, holidays, and travel. In this section we will provide training for how you can order from a restaurant menu using your *MAGIC-HAND*.

You may use the sample menu provided on the next page, or better yet, study the menu from one of your local restaurants if they will allow you to take one or try to find one published in your newspaper. In all situations you will be able to use your *MAGIC-HAND*, but it takes practice.

Imagine you are with a group of friends and it is nearing dinnertime, so you all decide to go out to eat. You still have 4 palm-portions and 1 thumb oil remaining for the day. How will you order? What will you eat?

There is more than one correct answer, but all answers must follow the guidelines of the *MAGIC-HAND* Eating Plan.

Go to the next page and pretend you are ordering now. Say:

"I will have ____

____

____".

It might be helpful to look at the dessert menu first so that you will know how many chits you can use for the meal.

If you are not having dessert, tell us how you will use your chits. Name the food. My:

Milk palm-portion is for ________________________________

Fruit palm-portion is for ________________________________

Carbohydrate palm-portion is for __________________________

Protein palm-portion is for ______________________________

Oil/fat thumb-portion is for ______________________________

Vegetables are ______________________________________

FULLY'S

APPETIZER'S

Peel and eat shrimp......... Crab stuffed mushrooms......
Calamari strips............ Sautéed mushrooms...........
Steamed artichoke.......... Chicken fingers............

SALADS

Caesar salad.............. Chicken Caesar............
(served with garlic bread)

PRIME RIB-STEAKS-RIBS

All dinner entrees served with your choice of homemade French onion soup or a garden salad, fresh baked bread and your choice of a baked potato, French fries, Rice pilaf or Spanish rice. Have an enjoyable evening.

Fully's prime rib (full cut)..............................
Fully's prime rib (half-cut)..........................
Porterhouse..
Filet Mignon...
New York Steak...

SHELLFISH, FISH & CHICKEN

Australian lobster- 1 tail................................
Alaskan King crab..
Shrimp scampi..
Breast of chicken (choice of teriyaki or BBQ sauce).........
Fresh fish of the day (white wine & lemon or garlic butter).

DESSERTS

Ice cream pie............. New York cheesecake.......

BEVERAGES

Coffee, tea .... Milk, buttermilk...........

Now imagine that you receive the order and visualize the food in front of you. How large are each of the portions? Describe.
To keep to palm-portion sizes, what food will be left on your plate?

____

____

What will you doggie bag?

____

If you decided to have dessert, tell us what palm-portion(s) if any, from the foods you previously named, will you need to give up.

____

What dessert will you order?

____

Is it likely to come in a palm-portion size?________________________________

Party pushers

Saying no to food is something most of us have not learned. Slim people seem to know when to stop eating and how to say no. Fat people generally eat too much and have difficulty saying no. We must learn the secrets of the slim people, and again it takes practice, because our old habits of accommodating our hosts, and of freely consuming all the food put in front of us need to be extinguished.

In this world there are people called "pushers". They push food on people. At a party they will say, "Have another piece." At dinner they will say, "You must have seconds."

Because of pushers you will need to learn how to become a "slim-sayer". The slim-sayer knows what to say to counter the pusher. The pusher considers the person on a diet to be a challenge. So, never tell the pusher you are watching how much you eat. That will only add fuel to the fire. Think of the phrases that thin people say. If you can, with another person, each trade roles, as a "pusher" and "slim-sayer", in the following exercise.

For Circle Group participation:

Play this "game" with a partner. You are at a relative's home. A feast is on the table. Everyone has brought a "special" dish. It is the pusher's job to get you to have some more food. It is the slim-sayer's job to politely refuse.

Supply the "pusher" statement:

____

____.

Supply the "slim-sayer" response:

____

____.

Now trade places with your partner and do the same exercise again. You can play this game as long as you like. Try to find the responses that feel comfortable to you. And remember even if someone pushes something on your plate, you don't have to eat it. "Push" it on to someone else's plate! (Preferably a man with a hollow leg.)

No-chit days

Your job has been to learn how to use the *MAGIC-HAND* Eating Plan for a lifetime of staying slim. But every job has some vacation time built in. Each day you start with 12 palm-portion chits and 3 thumb-portion chits. The program is absolutely livable. But, there are some times when you would really like **not** to count chits. Thanksgiving, for example, might be one day. On the program you are permitted nine days a year where you do not need to keep track of your chits. These are no-chits days and you should decide ahead of time what days they will be. This does not mean that you gorge yourself on the day; it just means you don't have to count or worry about palm-portion eating. In other words, you can enjoy your birthday, eat as much of what you want, and still stay on the program.

Go through the months of the year and think of the special occasions or holidays when you would like **not** to count chits. Remember that the reason you are monitoring your food intake is because you have a tendency to gain weight when left to your own devices. So, sorry, it can't be that every day is a no-chit day!

Think of the days during the year that are special days for you that might include a festive eating celebration. If you have more than nine, cut back some days. If you have less than nine, be aware that you have some "floating days" and then take a no-chit day for some other selected event. Our year starts in January, so let's begin.

Next to the month place the date of the occasion or name the holiday when you would like to use a no-chit day. Select nine days over the year.

Your "party planner" for the year:

January________________________	July__________________________
February_______________________	August________________________
March__________________________	September_____________________
April__________________________	October_______________________
May____________________________	November______________________
June___________________________	December______________________

If you have any days left over they are: Floating days=_____

Do you have a total of 9 days? Mark these days in your calendar as "No-chit days". I hope you will find as I have, that even on your no-chit days, because you have been so trained in how to eat during the year, you still think in palm-portions. Nevertheless it's nice to have a break once in a while, and it's also nice to get back to counting chits since we know it brings us the reward of good health and looks.

Nurture

N 8

● Point 8

What is "food" for my soul?

1. Name five things that you really enjoy doing.

2. If you haven't already, select one of the above that you can incorporate into your life now. How can you put this activity into your life on a regular basis?

3. Name one thing that you haven't done in a long time that really nurtures or pampers you.

What would have to happen for you to enjoy this now?

For stress reduction practice slow breathing

One of the best things you can do for yourself to relieve distress is to practice abdominal breathing. Take long deep breaths that fully distend your rib cage and abdomen; then exhale slowly through your mouth. When you are about to face a tense situation remember to pause and take at least three deep breaths. It may not solve the problem but it will help you to take care of yourself.

Practice slow breathing whenever you want to calm yourself or in preparation for and during meditation.

Try this exercise right now. Stand straight. Place one hand against the small of your back and the other on your abdomen. Breathe in slowly, as if you are filling a tank and allow your midsection to expand. Your hand should feel some movement. (If your shoulders move this is a sign of incorrect breathing.) As you exhale tighten the abdominal muscles and release the air through your mouth blowing the stress away. Tilt your pelvis slightly forward. When doing this exercise or any other where muscles are tightened and released, remember that the muscle is always tightened on the exhale (push the air out) and the muscle is relaxed on the inhale (fill up).

So, breathe in and fill the abdomen- relax the muscles.
Breathe out and tighten the abdomen- tighten the pelvic muscles.
To relieve stress and feel better practice abdominal breathing.
(Note: You will automatically breathe abdominally if you do this exercise while lying with your back flat on the floor.)

For Circle Group participation:

If you have never meditated or have never consciously allotted a time to be quiet, you can now experience this silence. You will need a comfortable chair to sit in. Place your feet on the floor and sit straight. If you'd like, remove your shoes. With a timer allow yourself ten (or twenty) minutes of silence. Close your eyes and continue to breathe deeply. Soft restful music can play in the background. Some people may giggle at first-- that's okay, or you might feel awkward with others around. Calm down, relax, breathe deeply and just do it. Sit quietly for ten minutes and push your thoughts away. Mainly concentrate on your breathing. It takes much practice to push all thoughts out of your mind so if they come, gently let them go, and push them away. See if you can simply "be" sitting on your chair in tune with the rhythm of your own breathing. During this meditation when you feel you are really relaxed, almost in a semi-sleep state, you may wish to imagine yourself losing five pounds. Keep taking five pounds off of your body and seeing yourself at a reduced weight until you reach your ideal weight. Repeat an affirmation: "I am now at my ideal body weight of _____." As the pounds leave and you see yourself slimmer, let go of the weight you no longer want or need. Send it away.

Are you comfortable? Are you ready? Silence begin.

For Circle Group discussion:

The experience of ten (or twenty) minutes of silence for some people is unsettling because disturbing thoughts that have been pushed down can surface. Eventually you will be able to resolve and push away recurring thoughts. Remember that the silence of meditation is healing. Your goal is to meditate each day for twenty minutes. This experience shows how long ten minutes of silence feels, and how restful it can be. Some people awaken from meditation feeling as if they have been on a restful "vacation".

What was your experience in these moments of silence?

____

____

____

When could you find the time to meditate on a daily basis?

____

Daily

● Point 9

A thumbnail sketch

The *MAGIC-HAND* Eating Plan offers you a hand-trick for keeping your weight under control. What you need to do is learn all the food groups that the fingers of your hand represent and understand that the finger food groups above the palm of your hand are measured in palm portion sizes. Your thumb measure is used for fats and oils. You are allowed twelve palm-portions and three thumb portions a day. Vegetables are unlimited. Every day is a new day. If for some reason you do not consume all of your chits they are not saved for the next day. Also if you go over your allotted chits one day, you do not hold back chits on the next day. Every day you get fifteen chits, twelve palms and three thumbs. So, every day is a new day on the *MAGIC-HAND* Eating Plan.

To stay motivated on this program for the rest of your life requires some self-knowledge. The following questions may not be easy to answer, but will help you discover what is really behind your desire for weight loss and control.

What are your reasons for losing weight? Why do you want to lose weight? Are these good enough reasons for a lifetime? *(List your reasons.)*

Can you picture yourself at your ideal weight? What difference will maintaining your ideal weight make in your life?

Are there any obstacles? Is there anything holding you back from achieving your ideal weight?

Are you able to say that you love yourself enough to invest in your own well-being?

The magic wand

The answers to the previous questions may make the difference between success and failure. For you to be successful you must stay with the program. Every day think of how nice it will be to fit into your ideal size clothes. You can mentally have that pleasure now while your body catches up with the image you have created.

We are all motivated by the principles of pleasure and pain. And we can approach weight loss through a positive or negative avenue or a combination of both. To be clear about your own reasons for controlling your weight think about what is truly supporting your desire. If we are in pain, physically or psychologically, because of being overweight, we will want to stop the pain-- to do something about our condition. If we are in pleasure and joy about ourselves, our feelings of good self-worth and self-esteem will direct us to take care of our bodies.

Is your desire for weight control to eliminate the pain of being overweight? If so, describe this pain.

____

____

Is your desire for weight control to acknowledge a love for yourself by taking care of your body? If so, what will be the benefit?

____

____

Finger-palm counters

Many people on the *MAGIC-HAND* Eating Plan have thought of creative ways to keep count of their 12 palms and 3 thumb daily portions. For example, some people use paper tear-offs to count their chits, others use a pencil check mark in their check registers, and some move coins from one pocket to another to count chits. Another has used clothespins. The most graphic presentation is to see your own hand on paper and to count your chits on the food group fingers each day.

For Circle Group discussion:

What are you using to count chits?

____

Are you strictly following the program or using modifications? Explain.

____

____

____

Once you have lost your weight, would you be tempted to go back to your old patterns of eating? If so, how can you motivate yourself to stay with the program?

____

____

____

Can you commit to living this way the rest of your life to maintain your ideal weight?

____

Now. Let's sing!

We've Got the *MAGIC-HAND* Eating Plan

(Sing to the tune of "He's Got the Whole World in His Hands")

We've got palm-portions in our hands
We've got finger food-groups in our hands
We've got a thumb measure in our hands
We've got the *MAGIC-HAND* Eating Plan

We've got a little-bit for Oils in our hands
We've got a Protein finger in our hands
We've got the Carbohydrates in our hands
We've got the *MAGIC-HAND* Eating Plan

We've got the Milk and Dairy in our hands
We've got a Fruit finger in our hands
We've got abundant Veggies in our hands
We've got the *MAGIC-HAND* Eating Plan

We've got our ideal body in our hands
We've got all the food groups in our hands
We've got thumb-palm measures in our hands
We've got the *MAGIC-HAND* Good Health Plan

Note: The original song, a "spiritual", was often sung with no music--hands softly clapping to the rhythm.

Appendix D

A Quick Thumb-Nail Sketch

You'll need thick paper, pen, and penny size magnets to create your personalized ***MAGIC-HAND***
(or use the sheet provided on the next page)

(1) **Write your first name** in the top left corner. Place your left hand palm down on the sheet of paper. Spread your fingers so there is enough room to trace between them. Now trace the outline of your hand using a pen.

(2) **Fingers represent food groups**: Write above the pinky, Milk & Dairy; write above the thumb Oils & Fats; write above the middle finger Carbohydrates; write above the index finger Protein; write above the ring finger Fruit. In the open space between thumb and index finger, write Vegetables.

(3) **The palm represents portion size**: Draw a broken circle as large as possible to fit inside the palm of your hand. This is your personalized palm-size portion.

(4) **Divide each finger into 3 joints** (to count the number of portions each day).

(5) **Place the drawing** on your refrigerator with 5 magnets in the center of the palm (You can make your own magnets by cutting out sections of a flat business or promotional card magnet.)

(6) **Each day**: You are permitted 3 palm-portions (no thicker than your thumb) or a cupped palm for each food group above the palm. You are permitted 3 thumb portions (thumb-size or to the knuckle joint) of Oils & Fats. All together you have 15 "chits".

(7) **Count** the palm or thumb portion consumed by placing the magnet on the finger food-group. After you have moved the magnet 3 times for each food group, you have used all of your allotted chits for the day. (Remember Vegetables are unlimited.)

(8) **You are permitted** 12 palm-portions and 3 thumb portions every day.

(9) **Laminate** your drawing if you want to keep it in place for the rest of your life!

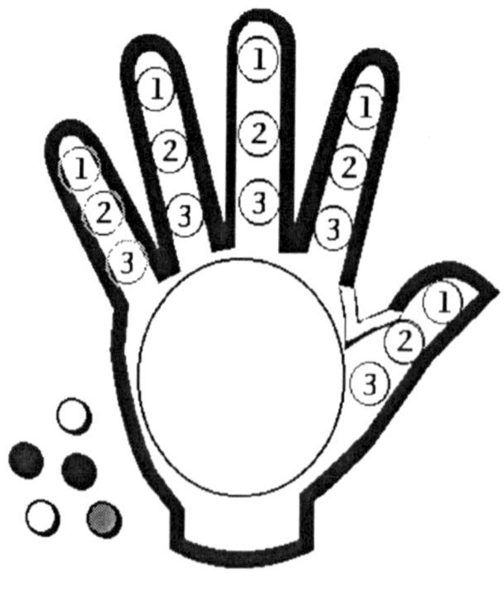

.........'s *MAGIC-HAND*®

...COPY THIS PAGE OR CUT ALONG THIS LINE. DRAW YOUR HAND. PLACE ON REFRIGERATOR WITH MAGNETS...

.......COPY THIS PAGE OR CUT ALONG THIS LINE.........

Appendix E

MAGIC-HAND Chits Page

Start With 21-Days

DAY	Milk&Dairy			Fruit			Carbs			Protein			Oils&Fats			Vegetables		
1																		
2																		
3																		
4																		
5																		
6																		
7																		
8																		
9																		
10																		
11																		
12																		
13																		
14																		
15																		
16																		
17																		
18																		
19																		
20																		
21																		

Place a checkmark in the box for each chit you use. If you go over your chit allotment place a "O" next to that DAY. Place a strike (/) through the DAY when you've completed or stayed within the allotted 12 palms, 3 thumbs. Vegetables are unlimited so you do not need to monitor. Column is included only as a reminder.

Keep Going 42 days

DAY	Milk&Dairy			Fruit			Carbs			Protein			Oils&Fats			Vegetables		
22																		
23																		
24																		
25																		
26																		
27																		
28																		
29																		
30																		
31																		
32																		
33																		
34																		
35																		
36																		
37																		
38																		
39																		
40																		
41																		
42																		

........COPY THIS PAGE OR CUT ALONG THIS LINE........

The 63-Day Challenge

DAY	Milk&Dairy			Fruit			Carbs			Protein			Oils&Fats			Vegetables		
43																		
44																		
45																		
46																		
47																		
48																		
49																		
50																		
51																		
52																		
53																		
54																		
55																		
56																		
57																		
58																		
59																		
60																		
61																		
62																		
63																		

Maintain for a lifetime of good health, happiness and weight control.

Keep Track in Your Checkbook Register!

Copy or cut out this weekly Chit Page to carry with you.

DAY	Milk&Dairy			Fruit			Carbs			Protein			Oils&Fats			Vegetables		
Mon.																		
Tues.																		
Wed.																		
Thu.																		
Fri.																		
Sat.																		
Sun.																		

Cut or fold over here.

DAY	Milk&Dairy			Fruit			Carbs			Protein			Oils&Fats			Vegetables		
Mon.																		
Tues.																		
Wed.																		
Thu.																		
Fri.																		
Sat.																		
Sun.																		

Cut or fold over here.

DAY	Milk&Dairy			Fruit			Carbs			Protein			Oils&Fats			Vegetables		
Mon.																		
Tues.																		
Wed.																		
Thu.																		
Fri.																		
Sat.																		
Sun.																		

Appendix F

Circle Groups

About the *MAGIC-HAND* Association

Knowing what to do, what foods to eat and how to monitor portions, is essential. However, a helping hand to maintain good lifestyle habits is often crucial for success. To this end the *MAGIC-HAND* Association assists Circle Groups to bring people together who are interested in mutual support. People like yourself can find or form a Circle Group by visiting the *MAGIC-HAND* Association website. The basics are given below:

How to Form a Circle Group

To form a Circle Group here are the steps to follow:
You will need to form a **T E A M**:

Three At Least	Participating members for the Circle Group
Experience	Knowing the *MAGIC-HAND* training course
Administrative	Registering the Circle Group with *MAGIC-HAND*
Meeting space	Providing a place to meet for Point sessions

Find a place to meet. This could be a person's home, meeting room, or restaurant. Establish a time when on a regular basis at least 3 people can attend. Eventually through word of mouth or notices others will join the Circle Group.
Select **Three Linking Rings**:

Ruling-Hand: Contact phone number and/or e-mail for the Circle Group.
Right-Hand: Assists the Ruling-Hand, may organize registration events.
Post-Hand: Meeting notices. Donations for Circle Group expenses.

Register your Circle Group with the *MAGIC-HAND* Association at the www.dranne.org or www.*MAGIC-HAND*.org website. Select a name for your Circle Group not to exceed nine letters. You will be asked to provide the Circle Group Name, Meeting Place & Zip code, Time, Day, Frequency you meet plus your Phone Number and/or e-mail address. In this way others can find you. After you register you will receive program updates and session guidelines.

What happens in the Circle Group

After the Circle Group is registered with the *MAGIC-HAND* Association, participants should plan to meet on a regular basis. Each participant brings her or his own copy of the *MAGIC-HAND* Eating Plan book. The MAGIC-SQUARE Card (found here on page F-3) is placed on the table with name facing out so that everyone can see your name. This is especially helpful when new people join the group.
The purpose of the Circle Group is to review each PRACTICE Point in the book, and then to keep repeating the Points thereby providing continuing support for the program.

These meetings are highly structured. The Circle Groups available from the *MAGIC-HAND* website have agreed to follow our guidelines and have access to downloadable materials necessary to operate the Group. The goal of the *MAGIC-HAND* Association is to provide these instructions to all Circle Groups so that the best possible results can be obtained. This program format design has been thoroughly tested. Each PRACTICE Point is designed to be covered in a 45-minute period, no more, no less. We aim for consistency in our Circle Groups and trust that our guidelines are followed. Check our website to make sure the Circle Group you are attending is registered.
So, this is what happens: you arrive at the meeting place for the Circle Group (on time) with your book. You sit down at a table, place your MAGIC-SQUARE card on the table, and place the book in front of you opened to the PRACTICE Point to be discussed. The MagiGuide, reads the Open statement, participants read paragraphs aloud as directed, the MagiGuide reads the Close statement, and the 45-minute Point session is ended.
Anyone participating in a Circle Group may contact the *MAGIC-HAND* Association through our website if there are any questions or concerns.

Who is the MagiGuide?

The MagiGuide is the person who leads the Circle Group for that Point session. It is the job of the MagiGuide to read the "Open" statement at the beginning of each meeting, and to direct the reading of PRACTICE paragraphs among participants. Questions and answers in the workbook are shared by the group. The Point session ends with the MagiGuide reading the "Close" statement. The role of the MagiGuide can be rotated among members of the Group so that different people may lead sessions if that is desired. Run your Circle Group with one person volunteering to be the MagiGuide to Open and Close the next Point session. This responsibility can rotate among Circle Group members.

Types of Circle Groups

The MagiGuide may be a **Volunteer,** or an **Independent** contractor or a **Member** of a club or organization that sponsors the Circle Group.
The Independent contractor may provide the program if she or he agrees to follow the program and fee guidelines. For some being able to charge for services while being a MagiGuide could be an avocation or full-time and very rewarding occupation.

Volunteer: Free of charge at a home, a place of business, or other.
Independent: Groups are guided by a professional or credentialed person.
Member: A club structure may be desirable for Circle Groups. Existing clubs or organizations may want to offer this program to their members.

Charges for services or memberships will vary depending on the type of Circle Group. Only persons with *MAGIC-HAND* Eating Plan materials are permitted to participate in Circle Group Point sessions. In general, new participants may enter at any Point.

Start at any Point until all Nine Points are completed.
Then continue to repeat Points as long as you want.

Cut out and then fold over:

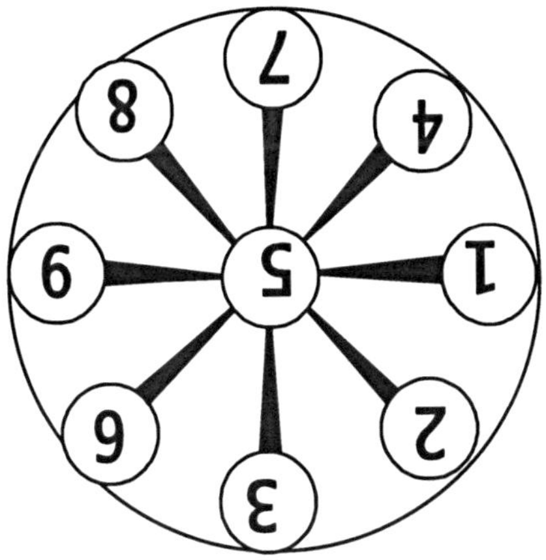

------- fold here

THE

MAGIC-SQUARE

for:

____

9 lifetime

Copy or cut out your MAGIC-SQUARE card to use at Circle Group meetings. Write your first name on the line above "9 lifetime". Make sure to fill-in the dot when you complete that Practice Point.

MAGIC-HAND Circle Groups

Below is a space for you to place a card or information about your local Circle Group.

Circle Group information:

Give a man a fish and you feed him for a day.

Teach a man to fish and you feed him for a lifetime.

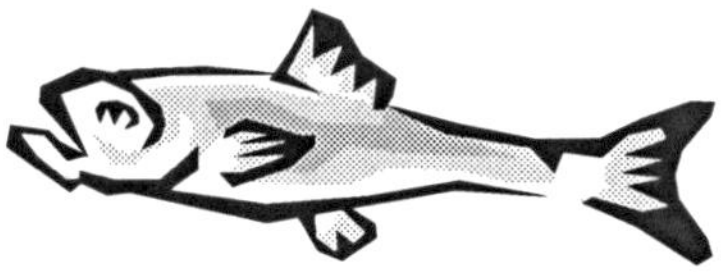

---Chinese proverb

Printed in the United States
43027LVS00001BA/31-58